BUCKET LIST
WEIGHT LOSS

• • • • • • • • • • • •

BY JAN MANNING

Table of Contents

Prologue v
My promises to you: vii
Chapter 1 - I am you.. 1
Chapter 2 - We are the true experts here 11
Chapter 3 - Changing Standards.. 15
Chapter 4 - The Yo-Yo Begins to Spin 27
Chapter 5 - A Change of Direction... 39
Chapter 6 - Life in Denial... 51
Chapter 7 - The Great Food Revolt 57
Chapter 8 - Hello, Scale!.. 63
Chapter 9 - How I Did It 69
   • BLWL *Concept 1*: "Four hours from now" 71
   • BLWL *Concept 2*: "Gut talk"... 74
   • BLWL *Concept 3*: "Handling depression" 81
   • BLWL *Concept 4*: "Hunger is good" 82
   • BLWL *Concept 5*: "Calorie tally"..................................85
   • BLWL *Concept 6*: "Weighing in" 93
   • BLWL *Concept 7*: "Move it" 103
   • BLWL *Concept 8*: "Tummy knows best"....................109
   • BLWL *Concept 9*: "Keep it real" 112
   • BLWL *Concept 10*: "Lose the clock" 114
   • BLWL *Concept 11*: "Water" 115
Chapter 10 - Q & A.. 121
An afterthought...for men only 139
Bucket List Weight Loss Recap 141
About the author.. 143

Prologue

Bucket List: The things you dream of accomplishing/ experiencing before you die. The things you don't want to have on your mind as "unfinished business" when your lights start to go out.

My promises to you:

- This diet will work where others have failed.

- You will feel healthier and look terrific.

- You don't necessarily have to give up your favorite foods.

- This diet is totally designed by you for your body.

- You can mess up once in a while!

- You will detoxify your body with this plan.

- You will achieve your Bucket List dream of being thin.

From the diary of a 15-year-old in 1968

Feb. 11

'I've eaten too much again, and I'm getting fat again too.'

Feb. 21

'I have starved myself for the last 3 days now, and I'm down to 134 at night. My goal is 130 by the end of the month, and then to 125 or below. I want to be SKINNY.'

March 12

'Since Mary D. challenged me to a weight losing contest, I've virtually quit eating til Thursday night. Thursday morning in gym class we'll weigh in.'

March 14

'Oh, Mary and I called off the contest last night, so I've been stuffing myself.'

March 27

'I have less than two weeks to 'shape up' and lose 10 lbs.'

July 18

'All I've been doing the past week is eating, and I'm trying desperately to get off the kick. I weigh so much now that I won't even put it down, because it's written in my mind. I must get down to 135 maximum in 1 or 2 weeks :'

August 13

'Starting tomorrow I'm going on a starvation diet for about a month till school starts. I've got to do something. I bet I could even model if I could get the figure! Others have said it too, and if that's not inspirational, I don't know what is!!'

Chapter 1

• • • • • •

I AM YOU

This is me:

I've been big all my life. Not obese. Just plain big. Now I'm small. Tall (5'10") and willowy.

I've worn sizes 12 to 16 almost all my adult life. I thought size 12 was the "right" size for me. Now I wear a size 4-6. In the S-M-L-XL world, I'm S. I didn't think my frame would allow me to get this small. I was wrong.

I used to wear a Size 40DD underwire bra that cost $55. Now I wear a 36C athletic bra that cost $15.

I yo-yo dieted all my life...until I developed my *Bucket List Weight Loss System.* Now I'll never be "big" again.

I lost 43 pounds in eight months with *BLWL,* and have effortlessly kept it off for two years

I eat real food.

I drink alcohol.

I no longer have cravings.

I no longer have intestinal gas.

I sleep well at night.

I feel 30 years younger than my actual age (60).

I may start a new career as a runway model.

I've undergone four total hip replacements since I was 40. Not a joint in my body is sore since I lost the 43 pounds.

My blood pressure and cholesterol are great!

My body looks good no matter what clothing I put on it.

I still occasionally eat and drink way too much of the wrong things.

I'm the thin one in most gatherings.

I will die having lived in my dream-size body.

I was just like you.

Now I'm going to tell you how you can be just like me.

But first, you're going to find out how similar your life and mine have been. We may have grown up in different environments, but we share common bonds and understandings that naturally thin people will never appreciate. As I guide you on a brief autobiographical journey into my life as a "large person," I hope you'll think back about the specifics of your own life. If weight has been an issue to you all your life, then you'll be able to identify with much of my story. That's the good news; that's why my *Bucket List Weight Loss* method will work for you too. You and I are very similar. And if I achieved my bucket list goal, you can too. *I encourage you to settle for nothing less than your biggest dream! It is absolutely attainable!*

Just so you don't think I'm attempting to pose as the next big weight-loss savior, nutritional expert or health guru, let's set the record straight. I'm not a professional on any of those subjects. You can find the "professionals'" books already out there in the stores. You'll be able to identify them right away, because the authors all have letters and titles after their names—PhD, MD, DO, PsyD, EdD, BFD or whatever. I don't have any letters after my name. I'm an average person who's had an average college education, lived an average life, and has carried an average 20 to 30 pounds of weight on her frame for most of her adult life. I am you. And I lost the extra weight once and for all.

Frankly, I've written this book for my own self-serving reasons:

1. It will remind me how I finally lost the extra weight I'd carried around since adolescence, and how I achieved a lifetime dream of being a Size 6. Having written it down, now I can refer back to it if I ever need to re-charge my motivation or confidence to maintain a Size 6 for life.

2. It will allow me to share this exquisite gift with you, knowing you can do the same thing I did. *Bucket List Weight Loss* is well within your grasp! And I'm not talking about going from a Size 16 to a Size 12 and calling it good. I'm talking about going the distance to a Size 6 or even a Size 4.

If you're over the age of 40 and have had it with dieting....if you want a way of eating that suits your own body and not someone else's...if you want to feel lighter, healthier, and twenty years younger....if one of the items on your "bucket list" is to become the size of your wildest, sexiest dreams....this book is for you. Being the size you really want to be is absolutely possible, and you can get there without pills, injections, food supplements or eating disorders. I did it, and so can you.

Your personalized method of *Bucket List Weight Loss* may turn out to be a bit different from mine. You may take issue with some of my theories, and you may come up with some modifications for your own plan. And that's fine. I don't care whether you drink Diet Coke or Diet Pepsi, whether you're conservative or liberal, whether you prefer baseball or football. We all follow separate paths to our goals because we are individuals. But I know you and I are more similar than we are different. You--like me--really *can lose all the weight you want*—and substantially more than you ever thought possible. You can enjoy the *freedom of being thin* for the first time in your life, and leave this world with that one little item ("I'd love to be a healthy Size 6") crossed off your "bucket list."

I really am you. That's how I know you're miserable being over-weight. I know you've struggled with self esteem issues and self confidence most of your life. I've seen you snacking in the car next to me when we're sitting at a stoplight, and you thought no one was watching. I've met you coming out of dressing rooms with arms full of clothes that "didn't quite work." I've seen you posing with coworkers for Christmas photo greeting cards, where the people on either side of you were skinny, and there you were, trying to hide your wide hips by standing a little behind them. I've watched you in yoga class, struggling to get comfortable in positions but hindered by rolls of fat around your stomach and hips.

I know your agony and your secret, most selfish wish: "If I could have anything I wanted right now, I'd be thin, because that would fix everything else that's wrong in my life." We don't like to admit our deepest wishes are that self-centered, but let's face it. If the genie popped out of the bottle right now and said she'd grant you one wish, you would probably ask to be thinner. After all, being thinner would fix just about every other problem we have, right?

Here's where I'm supposed to say, "Of course not!" and remind you that being thin is much less important than establishing world peace. But I'm not going to cave on this one. You're reading this book because the matter of losing weight, once and for all, *is* that important to you. And it should be. After all, losing weight and becoming thin has multiple life-enhancing benefits. And the more enhanced your life is, the more effective you can be in helping establish world peace.

Just think of the benefits you're about to experience.

1. No more achy joints

2. Greater self confidence

3. More energy

4. Better acceptance in society

5. Getting a better job

6. A better love life

7. Looking great in EVERYTHING you wear

8. Not having to hold your stomach in for every photo

9. Looking and feeling younger

10. Doing better in your chosen sports or recreational activities

Being branded since birth as a "big-boned" Scandinavian, I learned to accept being bulky. I didn't think it was physically possible for me to become small without suffering from anorexia or cancer. I was wrong. At age 59, I melted the excess fat off my 5'10" body and discovered a basic, normal-size skeletal frame that wasn't bulky at all. The frame was covered with well defined muscle that had been camouflaged under layers of fat. My "big-ness" had been from sheer fat, not bone or muscle. What was once a Size 16 body became a Size 6. The skeletal structure hadn't changed a bit, I'd just shed the fat layer.

For the first time in my life, my dream of weight loss and body change has come true. Completely. Permanently. The fear of gaining it back is gone, because I know how to live and eat like a healthy Size 6. Never again will I be called an "amazon." Never again will I be taunted and called "Moose," as I was in high school. The emotional pain of being big, and the obsession with food and its consequences, are blessedly gone from my life, freeing me to use my energy on much more creative and altruistic endeavors!

No, there aren't any fancy letters, titles or degrees hanging on the end of my last name. But I am an expert on how I lost the weight and performed a life-changing miracle on myself. If you take issue with my methods and my philosophy, don't bother sharing your concerns with me. This is my story, my discovery, my journey. Just remember.....*I am you.* So just maybe the road map I'm about to give you will lead you to the same destination.

By the way, I turned 59 in 2011. At my birthday dinner, I wore size 6 black leather pants and a hot pink, fuzzy, short-waisted sweater. I looked great and felt even greater. No fat rolls or bulges anywhere. The clothes felt fabulously comfortable—not tight or binding or too small. The body beneath them didn't hurt anywhere either. The hip and knee joints were pain-free, rejoicing that nearly 40 pounds had been lifted off them over the past several months.

Truly, I never imagined I'd reach this goal, this peace-with-food-and-with-myself state of euphoria. I never planned that at age 59 I'd finally have the figure of a runway model. I'd anticipated my dying thoughts on this earth would be something like, *"Thank you for a good life, Lord, take care of my husband and the dogs, I'm so grateful for a good life, although I do wish I'd lost that weight and found out what it was like to be skinny, but...oh well...."*

Yup, losing my extra fat was a "bucket list" item, something I dreamed of accomplishing before I died, but not something I really thought I'd attain.

Now, here I am, feeling 30 years younger than my age. Stronger. Agile. Clear-headed. I can bound up stairs again. My concentration's better. I run my hands over the body that was once coated in several extra inches of fat. Now I feel the body...the bones, muscles, tendons, my femoral artery. It's almost like studying skeletal anatomy in high school biology class. I can actually see what strings me together. I can feel muscles and ligaments flexing. All this time, there was actually a BODY beneath that lard. At long last, I've met and seen the wonderful structure that's worked so hard to carry me through this life.

Whenever I'd lost weight in the past on one diet program or another (as we all have), I' d live with a silent dread of knowing that if I stopped drinking the liquid shakes, started eating carbohydrates again, or started eating "normally," I'd gain back the weight I'd lost. And it happened every time. That dread is now gone, partly because I have this book to remind me of how easy it was to lose 40 pounds and how equally easy it is to keep it off forever, with a new way of eating.

After I lost 40 pounds in eight months of *Bucket List Weight Loss*, and shrunk from a Size 12 to a Size 6, friends started pumping me for details about my method.

"What happened?" "How did you do it?" "What program were you on?" Weight Watchers? Atkins? South Beach? Jenny Craig? Nutrisystem? Mackeral Pudding? When I told them I hadn't followed a "program" or diet, their jaws would drop a little lower, and they'd stand there in silence, waiting for more explanation. Until now, I've just been smiling and saying, "I'm writing a book about it."

Knowing how many other people can benefit from my incredible bucket list experience, I feel an obligation to share how I did it. You will appreciate this story and method if you have ever...

...hated yourself for being the weight you are.

...been bullied, tormented, or just felt self conscious about your size.

...been as obsessed with thoughts of food as you are with your weight.

...dieted successfully and then gained it back (with a few extra pounds added).

...felt hopeless, helpless and powerless over food and your weight.

...avoided the scale to remain in denial of your weight fluctuations.

...stayed home from a social function because, at the last minute, you couldn't find anything that fit.

...sworn that you'd go on a starvation diet if it killed you.

...ignorantly and secretly envied anorexics.

...labeled chapters of your life according to what diet you were on at the time.

...hated yourself for being so self-obsessed.

Good grief, what a heavy mental load we carry along with our extra poundage! Shedding the pounds also means shedding that energy-draining emotional burden. It's time to stop kicking yourself. It's time for you to stop crippling your body with the extra weight and your mind with the self-loathing. Go ahead and realize your dream, as I did mine. Go ahead. Become a Size 6. It's a totally obtainable dream. Stay a Size 6. That's even better.

You won't do it, though, if you accept your current size, give up, or say, "Screw it, I'm fat and it's okay because so is everyone else these days."

You won't do it by rationalizing that life is short and you should enjoy as much pasta, ice cream and nachos as you like.

You won't reach your goals if you give up and say, "Obviously I was never meant to be slim. It's physically impossible for me to get down to a Size 6".

You will only reach your *Bucket List Weight Loss* if you start to believe in yourself and your ability to do this. And you must start at once so you have that much longer to enjoy the miracle you're about to perform on your own body.

Chapter 2

• • • • • •

WE ARE THE TRUE EXPERTS HERE

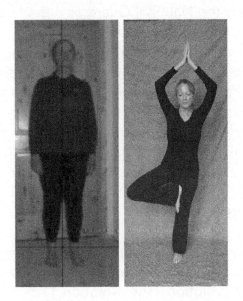

There's nothing special about the reasons I gained weight. I have no good excuses. No medical conditions, no parental abuse, no pregnancies—nothing but a comfy, complacent childhood in northern Minnesota, where supper usually consisted of some form of fried meat and boiled potatoes.

My home life was akin to "Father Knows Best." (For those of you too young to remember, that was an old sitcom featuring a working dad, a stay-at-home mom, and three nicely behaved kids. Today people criticize it for portraying the American family in a too-good-to-be-true, harmonic, idealistic light. Like it or not, our family was closer to that picture than to "Married With Children" or any more "contemporary" sitcom.)

In school I liked creative writing, music, and my boyfriend. At 5'10", I was the tallest girl in my 1970 high school graduating class. In college I studied communications and got a bachelor's degree. Following graduation, I held a variety of marketing and media jobs, joined the National Guard as a public affairs officer, did some freelance magazine writing, and worked as a journalist in the country music industry. Later in life, I changed directions and became a dog trainer with a very successful small business. Throw in some stints as a professional bartender, magazine editor, and dog food distributor, and you have an odd mix of experience that has little to do with health and fitness. I did write a couple articles on weight training and backpacking for Cosmopolitan, and I worked part-time as a fitness instructor at a YMCA for a few months. But that's the extent of my professional experience in the field of dieting and exercise.

However, I'm a bona fide expert on diets, just like you are. In fact, you and I probably have read the same books over the years— Dr. Atkins Diet Revolution, The Rotation Diet, The Complete Scarsdale Medical Diet, The Setpoint Diet, The South Beach Diet, Ultimate Weight Loss Solution. We also know that every one of them will work, if followed. We know that because we've tried them all, at least for short periods of time. We also know each diet stops working as soon as we stop following it. Worse than that, we know our weight rebounds with a vengeance. The dreaded diet yo-yo.

So if you and I are alike, and if neither one of us is a medical professional, why should you listen to me? Because I found the answers to a problem that hits us both on such an emotional level that it permeates every facet of our lives. I've found secrets to successful and permanent weight loss. That makes me more of an expert than you, but it also makes me someone with whom you can relate. The weight-loss professionals will sell you programs, provide you with pre-packaged foods, and tell you what to eat to lose the weight. But they don't tell you what to do when you leave the program or return to "normal" eating. What I'm about to teach you is as "normal" as eating can get. There's no program or products to purchase. You will be encouraged to change a few simple habits, and to form a new relationship with your body. You'll develop better listening skills and become more conversant with your body. You'll learn to rethink "hunger" and to embrace it rather than feed it.

I thought permanent weight loss was out of my reach, but it wasn't. *Because you and I are alike, you can reach your dream weight too, and maintain it for the rest of your life.*

Chapter 3

● ● ● ● ● ●

CHANGING
STANDARDS

Somewhere in a closet, I have a big box of home movies on 8-millimeter reels. That's what we used back in the '50s and '60s. No sound (except the clacking and whirring of the projector we used) poor color, and lots of wild, unedited shots of sky and grass. My mom wryly named one of the reels, "The Well Fed Family." It starred all five of us—mom, dad, and three kids—playing around the dock and beach at our summer lake cabin in northern Minnesota. We all filled out our swimsuits with more than ample flesh.

Ironically, if somebody transposed those five people into a present-day digital video, they probably wouldn't even look chunky. Not by today's standards. They'd be thinner than most of America's currently young families.

Modern society has allowed its standards of appearance and personal behavior to slide. We hear about rampant obesity in the U.S. and we see it every day, but if you travel to other developed and westernized countries, you'll see the same trends. What the hell happened? It's as if everyone just gave up and said, "Okay, it's easier to be fat, so let's just make that the acceptable norm."

People don't even try to hide their fat rolls anymore. You can't go anywhere now without seeing young women, in particular, who seem to flaunt their adipose tissue, letting their muffin tops hang out over their pants. They draw attention to their fat with tattoos that peak out from under skin-tight tops defining every dimple of cellulite. Personally I find this "in your face" slovenliness revolting, and I don't think it's just because I was born in 1952 in northern Minnesota.

Granted, fat people just weren't as common when I was growing up. Kids were more active; they played outside after school and all day long in the summer. They ate fewer processed foods, and there wasn't a MacDonald's or Burger King on every corner. People ate at home, usually sitting down to meals together. People dressed more modestly and did everything possible to hide fat rolls around their middles, fat bulges on their hips and backs, and flab on their arms. No one—not even skinny girls or the high school whores--wore skin-tight tops (spandex hadn't been popularized yet), and the only people with tattoos were old sailors. Skin exposure was limited to bare limbs in summer, or to modest bikinis for swimming.

You never wore low-cut tops revealing the crease between your breasts, and you would have died before exposing the crack between your butt cheeks when you bent over in hip-hugger pants. As you got dressed each day, you checked for bulges and lines, and changed your clothes if you found any in the full-length mirror. A respectable woman literally wouldn't leave her house without a girdle. "Tent dresses" were popular because they hid a multitude of sins. No one could be sure what was going on, fat-wise, underneath a baggy, shapeless A-line dress. They were great equalizers of fat and skinny women.

My mom sewed most of my school clothes—not from economic necessity but because she was creative and she enjoyed it—and I had a wonderful wardrobe of loose-fitting dresses that camouflaged my wider-than-standard hips and amply budding breasts. On a lark one day she ordered me a novelty dress she saw advertised in a newspaper ad. It was a disposable paper tent dress made from Yellow Pages! Thinking back, it was probably made of a hearty Tyvek-type paper material, although this was 1968 and Tyvek wasn't even around then. Anyway, even the skinny little model in the ad looked absolutely shapeless in this thing, as was the intention. Everyone already knew what you had underneath, and I think it was the mystique of "knowing but not seeing" that aroused the opposite sex. It certainly worked for my boyfriend. The paper dress barely stayed intact through one date.

A few years after the tent dress craze came loose-fitting tunics (that hid hips) and the shorter smock tops (that hid bellies). Actually, they both resembled maternity tops. I remember going shopping with a high school girlfriend, who was wearing a smock top over her huge boobs. A sales clerk came up to her and said, "When are you due, honey?" She never wore the top again. The irony? Today's clingy pregnancy fashions accentuate the belly bump, and even the non-pregnant women still look pregnant because of their fat stomachs. Honestly, I can't tell who's pregnant and who isn't anymore, and it's not because they're hiding it; it's because they're letting everything hang out!

There were about 300 kids in my high school class, and I only recall three or four chubs of each gender. Grade school classes were even leaner. From first through sixth grades, we had only one "fat girl" in the whole school. Poor Roberta would fit right in with today's school kids, but in 1960 she was considered fat.

No doubt she was stigmatized for life by the cruel teasing of her classmates.

Jack LaLanne, TV's first exercise guru, was a fixture in our living room every morning. During the summer I'd sit on the floor in front of the black and white TV and watch him do jumping jacks in his one-piece, stirrup-footed suit. Even to a nine-year-old, he was engaging and inspirational. He had my mom and me both convinced that shapeliness and vitality were found in a shakerful of whatever vitamin drink he was selling. Plus, he had two huge white German Shepherds, neither of whom seemed particularly intelligent or trained, but I liked to watch their cameo appearances at the beginning and end of each show. Jack LaLanne was one of my first heroes.

Back then, women didn't lift weights. They didn't jog. There were no co-ed health clubs. There were no high-profile varsity sports for girls, other than cheerleading. Women were supposed to be soft and yielding, not muscle-bound and strong. Women didn't sweat; they were supposed to simply "glisten." That totally ruled out any participation in cardio workouts (another term that hadn't yet been invented). So Jack LaLanne had the women's fitness market sewn up. Housewives exercised in the privacy and sanctity of their own living rooms. Old Jack was the only man they'd allow to watch them. It was a pretty intimate relationship. A daily workout consisted of 10 jumping jacks, 10 toe touches, and 10 repetitions of overhead presses, using cans of peas. Then there was the secondary workout you could get by shaking up his mixed drink in a cocktail shaker.

"You want that flabby underarm fat to disappear?" he'd challenge. "Just shake this for 30 seconds, and then—" he'd uncap the shaker and pour a frothy liquid into a tall glass, "enjoy one of these wonderful, delicious vitamin drinks." It was probably the original "meal replacement drink."

With Jack's help, my mother battled her own weight demons. She was chronically 10 to 15 pounds over her "ideal" weight. Again, by today's standards her 5'6" frame would have been considered fairly slim. But she honestly was a bit pudgy and she wasn't happy about it. My dad was an executive, and my mom felt a self-imposed pressure to maintain a standard of appearance that she thought was appropriate for a corporate exec's wife.

A few years ago I was paging through her tattered cookbook bible, "The Joy of Cooking," and found some notepaper tucked into the Calorie Chart page.

Breakfast:
½ c. orange juice
Poached Egg
Dry toast
Coffee

Lunch:
Salmon salad
Beef Boulion
Tea

Dinner
Dry martini
4 oz. beef
½ cup potatoes
Green salad
Total calories: 920

Poor woman. I feel sad for her now when I read her scribblings. I empathize with her, not as a daughter but as another woman. When I was a child, she always looked just fine to me. She was Mummy, smoking a cigarette as she talked to her galfriends on the phone or sat at a bridge table with them. She was firm and fairly shapeless around the middle, but only because of the ever-present girdle. My mother never lost the extra weight she so despised, until she got cancer when she was in her mid-50s. Like so many cancer patients, she withered to a jaundiced skeleton and died at age 57. She was a smoker, but pancreatic cancer is what did her in.

My brother and sister were seven and eight years older than I, respectively. My brother never had a weight problem till late in life, but my sister began her own struggles during adolescence. She loved to eat and she loved to cook, though my mom never gave her many opportunities in the kitchen, which was her domain. Because of my sister's growing weight problem, my mom all but banished her from the kitchen except to eat meals. So my sis made up for it any time our parents left us alone at home for a few hours. The minute their car pulled out of the garage, Sis was rummaging through the kitchen cupboards to see what she could throw together and devour before they returned. She came up with exotic concoctions like cocktail shrimp, horseradish and ketchup, and loved to bake Chef Boy Ar-Dee pizzas that came as a kit in a cardboard box. She'd sprinkle Nestle's Quick on vanilla ice cream, or whip up some oyster stew with canned oysters and condensed milk.

"Mmmmmm, here, try this," she'd say as she offered me a spoonful of whatever she'd invented. Most of the time I turned up my nose at it. But I did learn by watching. I learned that secret, forbidden eating was great recreational activity that could begin as soon as parents left the house. It was fun and adventurous, and of course we had to consume all the evidence before parents returned. I learned to eat Nestle's Quick straight off a spoon, and to enjoy peanut butter straight from the jar, without bread.

By the time I was in high school, weight had become an issue with me too. I was tall and pretty, but "big." Not fat, just big. As sexual hormones started raging, I packed on a few more pounds. I suppose a psychologist would call it sexual repression or something. I'd come home from an innocent date with my sweet boyfriend and make a beeline for the refrigerator before going to bed. After an evening of "making out" in his car (kissing, and nothing more), a pre-bedtime snack helped me unwind. Ice cream was the best, but one night I discovered frozen orange juice concentrate and used that as a substitute. I never considered that a can of frozen OJ concentrate contained 440 calories and enough sugar to keep me buzzing till morning.

The pounds continued to creep onto my butt and thighs. When I was 15, I started obsessing about my weight, my size, and food. I was 5'9" and over 140 pounds now, and none of it was solid because girls didn't "work out" back then. Despite my bigness I was well proportioned and had beautiful long auburn hair. My friends would say, "You're so tall…you should be a model." I began fantasizing about doing just that, even though I was already fifteen pounds too heavy for such a job.

In 1968, the term "supermodel" hadn't yet been born. They were just plain "models." The word was synonymous with a few tall, lanky beauties like Jean Shrimpton, Colleen Corby, and Penelope Tree. Later on the list expanded to include Gerry Hall, Cybill Shepherd, Imam, and Cheryl Tiegs. Every issue of Seventeen magazine included an ad for "Barbizon School of Modeling."

Their killer slogan: *"Be a model or.... just look like one."* The mere idea of looking like a model was enough to make any teenage girl drool...especially if she already had the height and potential looks, and I did.

My quest to be a model was a very secret dream; I dared not tell anyone outright. My mother would have had a cow and told me how foolish I was to even think of such a career. Others might say, "What a joke! Otteson thinks she could be a model! She's too fat. She's not cute enough." So, to avoid rejection on the home front, I kept my fantasy private. As long as I didn't actually pursue a modeling career, I wouldn't have to face the rejection on any level. But I could continue to dream, albeit unrealistically, that if I just lost fifteen pounds I could actually break into the business.

So there I was at 16—with raging hormones, all this height, an unobtainable fantasy that demanded I get skinny, and already a history of compulsive eating. It was a wonder I didn't become anorexic or bulemic. Those were not household terms back then, but of course the conditions they define had been around forever. I do believe if I'd known what anorexia and bulemia were, I would have been drawn toward them, much as copycat criminals are drawn to the dark side.

September 12, 1968

I have to write this right now quick before my steam simmers down. I'm sick and tired of having to think so much about food, and tired of thinking of what a big seat I have, and my hips!! And so help me, this is the last day I'm going to go through it, I swear on a stack of Bibles. I got it in 3 good blows today. The first was in Duluth, where, as usual, all the really CUTE clothes stopped at size 13. And

> if it wasn't for my bottom half I could easily wear 13 or 12. I fool myself into thinking it's just my height, but models don't wear 15s. No. 2 was tonight when Keith [boyfriend] said his mom said I sure was big! Well, of course she meant mostly tall, but I know. And I REFUSE to be compared to an Amazon. And I want people to be able to say to Keith, 'Boy, she sure is tall and thin.' No. 3 came when Mum had to alter a pattern for a vinyl jumper, and she had to add two inches to the hips. Even if I have to have a nervous breakdown, I'm not going to stay the size I am now. Even if I have to eat my hair or my fingernails, THIS IS THE END!"

What a sad entry this was into my teenage diary! Already the pain and obsession was there. Trying on new clothes that didn't fit. Loathing my own shape. Hearing my boyfriend's mother refer to me as "big" and failing to convince myself it was a euphemism for "tall."

I fantasized about being thin, threatened self mutilation (*"if I have to eat my hair or my fingernails"*) and felt willing to jeopardize my health (*"even if I have a nervous breakdown"*), just for weight loss. I wasn't about to actually act on any of these threats, nor did I have any sensible plan for losing the weight. Much of the pain I felt was probably hormonal, since the mood swings of self-loathing never lasted long enough for me to eat my hair or nails or have a "nervous breakdown." But the mood swings also caused me to eat more. Food was my immediate comfort. It's hard enough to set long-term goals when you're an adult, let alone a teenager unable to visualize anything past Friday night.

In 1970, during my senior year in high school, my boyfriend broke up with me, on orders from his parents who feared I'd end up pregnant. I was utterly devastated. I didn't want to live. I re-treated into my own shell, stayed at home, and ate because food was my nonjudgmental friend. It kept me company, and it never rejected me.

I gained another five pounds before graduation. School became a nightmare to me. A gang of popular girls in the junior class began bullying me for kicks. They were happy I'd broken up with my cute boyfriend and returned him to the open market. They expressed their joy by following me in the school hallways and chanting, *"Moose…Moose….Moose."* When they'd manage to find me alone in a restroom or science lab, they'd whisper, point, and giggle in an effort to make me paranoid. I'd pretend to ignore them, but I went home each night feeling like I'd rather die in my sleep than return to school the next day.

The real reason they chose me to terrorize? I'll probably never know. But at that vulnerable time in my life, I just assumed it was my size they were ridiculing. After all, why else would they chant *"Moose"* when they saw me?

My mom let me go shopping alone for the graduation outfit I'd wear under my cap and gown. I fell in love with a decidedly feminine white dress that buttoned up the front and had a fairly full, gathered skirt. It was a Size 13 and it barely fit me. I still remember the strain of buttons across the bustline and the waistline that was too tight, especially on that hot graduation night. My mom knew the dress was too small, but she let me wear it anyway. I got two presents from my folks that night. One was a lovely little diamond ring they'd had reset just for me. The other was a six-month membership to the "European Health Spa," a new exercise club that had just opened in Duluth, which was about twenty miles from our house.

Commercial spas and health clubs were relatively new concepts in 1970. The Duluth club was typical. The entryway was gaudily decorated with fake statuary, plastic ferns and fountains. The interior was supposed to look opulent with its red carpeting and heavily mirrored walls. The place stunk of sinus-clearing eucalyptus and chlorine bleach. The staff--skinny women in tight shorts and tops-- floated around the room, helping fat, inept women operate the various resistance machines. There wasn't a treadmill in the place. Elipticals, ski machines, stair steppers, and swiss exercise balls didn't exist in those days. But there were several "belt massagers," and they were always occupied. After all, the belt machine didn't require any kind of a workout. All you had to do was lean against this vibrating belt that circumnavigated your hips, and let it shake the fat off you. Of course all it actually did was make you itch. Maybe the scratching that came later was supposed to be part of the exercise routine.

I needed any exercise I could get to offset the calories I was ingesting. I discovered how easy it was to eat without restraint, now that I was driving myself and becoming more independent of my mother. I started college that fall in Duluth, moved into the dorm, and discovered that tater tots were available twelve hours a day in the cafeteria! During my freshman year of unbridled freedom, I partied, occasionally studied, attended most classes, ate pizza, charburgers and tater tots, and packed on about 15 pounds.

My dream of becoming a model faded into obscurity. I was maturing and learning to accept realities. Now a college student, I was becoming too old to start such a career. At 180 pounds, I'd have been too big even for plus-size modeling, if they'd even had such a thing back then. So I dedicated myself to a new, tangible career path: communications, which included radio, television production, and journalism. I'd found my niche, and finally college classes became more fun than partying. Editing the college newspaper, working in the radio station, and holding down a part-time job at the local TV station consumed a lot of energy I'd formerly put into food and weight issues. I was busy and happy, and my weight finally stabilized.

Chapter 4

• • • • • •

THE YO-YO BEGINS
TO SPIN

Pick a year in your life and recall a milestone from it—a moment or event defines that whole year for you. Many people would remember a year for the birth of a child, graduation from college, death of a close family member, or a surgery.

Chronic dieters, however, will tell you the weight-loss program they were following at the time, and they'll be able to tell you what size they wore on June 3 or October 21 of any given year.

1976. I joined the National Guard and went to basic training in Alabama. Weighed in at 176 pounds of flab and was issued Size 18 uniforms. Twelve long weeks later I'd firmed down to 162 pounds and had to trade the uniforms in for Size 14s. In basic training we had little time to eat, let alone sleep. Our appetites were down anyway, due to the stress, heat and humidity of spring at Ft. McClellan, Alabama. We did lots of PT (physical training) and marching. Every muscle was sore all the time. And there was that constant humiliation of lining up to be weighed every Monday morning. The consequences for gaining weight: pushups and humiliation dished out by our training officers in front of our peers. Losing that weight was easy, because we had virtually no choice.

Lesson eventually learned: Structure is good for all of us. How many times have you envied a well cared-for dog, who gets fed the same amount at the same times every day, and lacks opposable thumbs that would gain him entry to the fridge and the cookie jar? He has no choices and no temptations (other than the food we leave on the counter...or your expensive leather boots).

With structure, we physically and emotionally limit our thoughts and actions. Structured eating means we only have the opportunity to eat certain foods at certain times. This differs from "disciplined eating," which requires us to practice restraint. Structured eating may be a great way to start losing weight, but, because we're free-will creatures bombarded with temptations, we ultimately need to incorporate disciplined eating to keep it off.

1977. With basic training behind me, I returned to civilian life and "weekend warrior" status in the National Guard and Army Reserve. As reservists we met one weekend a month and two weeks every summer, during which we'd have to pass physicals, get weighed, and take a physical training test. A lot of reservists had "part-timer" attitudes back then, meaning they got overweight and out of shape since they were civilians 28 days a month. At testing time, lots of soldiers' weights and PT test scores were fabricated by record-keepers because it was easier for them to pass unit inspections that way. I fell in with all the other backsliders and gained back the weight I'd lost in basic training, plus some. The YoYo Syndrome had begun.

I moved to Nashville that year and landed a fantastic job as a writer with a country music magazine. Work days were fun, and nights were even better. All I could afford was canned soup for dinner, but I supplemented it at night with beer in the bluegrass bars I frequented, and typically topped off each evening with a few hot, fresh Krispy Kreme donuts to eat on the way back to my apartment. Krispy Kremes were available on every other street corner and were open all night. On the alternate street corners were "Krystal Burger" drive-ins, also open all night and peddling cheap food that slid down easily on top of several beers. I also discovered the southern delicacy of sausage and biscuits, which the editor's daughter would deliver to us about once a week in an aromatic sack straight from Jo-Jo's Biscuit Barn. My weight climbed to an all-time high of 192.

Lesson eventually learned: Don't eat just because everyone else is. If coworkers bring in a box of donuts or a bag of biscuits to share with the staff, just think of how much fatter they'll all be tomorrow. Be different! Be slimmer! Enjoy the aroma of the goodies; in fact, inhale deeply, and get your pleasure from your olfactory senses rather than from masticated globs of dough sliding down your throat and landing like a brick in your stomach.

Lee, our magazine's managing editor, recalls the first time he ever saw me back in early 1977. I'd dropped in to the publishing offices to apply for a job, and was sitting in the waiting room when he came back from lunch and glanced at me on his way down the hall to his office.

"All I remember about you was that you were wearing something red and you were BIG," he says, in his characteristically undiplomatic way. Well, I was.

In fact, I was so big—a true size 18 now—that I stayed home from several after-hours music functions because I was ashamed of myself and had nothing to wear. One night I was supposed to attend a prestigious showcase featuring a new, up-and-coming singer. Tickets for things like that were always free for those of us in the press. When it was finally time for me to leave my apartment for the showcase venue, I still hadn't found anything appropriate to wear. I combed my closet for something, anything, that would look good enough on me. *Nothing fit.* I sobbed, screamed, and swore at the body I'd developed, and the person I hated. I punished myself by staying home and having a pity party. I vowed things would change if it killed me, and that I'd start a starvation diet the next day.

"Going hungry and not eating can't possibly be any worse than feeling like this!" I swore to myself in preparation for the next day's diet. That left me the rest of the night to indulge, so I went to the late-night supermarket to get a Mrs. Smith's Boston Cream Pie. It would be the last, I promised to myself as I dove into it. But of course it wasn't.

1978. Ah, that was the year of the Stillman Diet, the second time around. The first time had been back in the early '60s when Dr. Stillman's low-carb, low-fat method was first introduced as "The Doctor's Quick Weight Loss Method." My mom had pounced on that one back then—after having limited success with the "Hollywood Diet," the "Grapefruit Diet" and the "Eat, Drink and Be Healthy Diet." Lo and behold, Stillman worked for her. She dropped about 12 pounds in 10 days. It even worked for me, a teenager...at least, for the short time I stuck with it. I dropped about seven pounds in a few days by eating lots of cottage cheese, canned tuna, hard-boiled eggs and sugar-free Jello. The Stillman diet was an extreme forerunner to modern-day Atkins. Unlike Atkins, however, it was touted as a fast, temporary fix and not a lifelong way of eating. Dr. Stillman warned that the common weight loss of seven to 15 pounds in the first week would reverse itself as soon as carbohydrates were re-introduced. His advice to followers was to follow a healthful, reduced-calorie diet to maintain the weight they'd lose on his extreme plan.

That's where most dieters, like my mom and me, fell down on the job. We could count calories all right, but we couldn't every get satisfied. We thought counting calories meant you ate lots of carrots and celery, and other low-calorie foods that you normally wouldn't consume in the first place—at least not in quantities. Poached chicken breast? Broiled cod? Steamed broccoli? Not popular in our house! So eating them as part of a restricted-calorie diet was an abnormal pain that only left us craving "real" food. The concept of indulging in a Peanut Buster Parfae at 730 calories, and then making up the allowed daily difference with more healthful food, was unthinkable, even though that PBP probably would have satisfied us and kept us from craving any-thing else high in calories for two days. The absolutely brilliant "Weight Watchers" philosophy of "Eat whatever you want, but in moderation" hadn't yet been commercialized. So the weight my mom lost on Stillman had come back. Plus a few more pounds. So had mine.

Lesson eventually learned: Eat what truly satisfies you, and you'll end up eating less overall. If you want a cookie, have a cookie. In fact, have two, followed by a huge glass of water. Eating a carrot when you really want a cookie will only make you angry and resentful, which will probably lead to eating ten cookies an hour later.

But in 1978, when I was desperate to lose weight, all I remem-bered about Stillman was the rapid weight loss. Five to seven pounds in two days? Who wouldn't be enticed to try it again? After all, when we're fat and unhappy, we think the *only* thing that can make us happy again is to change our bodies immediately. "I can't stand to be fat another minute," we shriek to ourselves. "I must be thin *tomorrow*. At the very least, I must drop ten pounds in two weeks. Then my life will be better." We find comfort in that thought...so much comfort that we might even head back to the kitchen and grab a cookie to celebrate.

The ads for weight-loss programs, which appear in newspapers every November (a precursor to the expected holiday weight gain) make us believe such overnight transformation is actually possible.

"Drop 25 pounds by New Year's!" "Go from a size 14 to a size 8 in four weeks!" "Start the program today, and be 15 pounds lighter in three weeks!"

Illustrating the ads are "before" and "after" photos of folks who've supposedly had success with the programs. The "before" usually shows some slovenly dressed, depressed-looking fat person slouched against a drab wall. The "after" shows the same person, supposedly, dressed to the nines and gleefully striking an "I'm too sexy for my clothes" pose. And this transformation all took place in a matter of weeks.

No wonder we program ourselves for fast results and failure. Just before Thanksgiving the ads say, "Lose 15 pounds by Christmas," and we start to believe it can actually happen. Not that it can't. Rapid weight loss is attainable through extreme measures, and when we're fat we don't care how extreme the measures may seem. All we can think about is losing 40 pounds by tomorrow morning when we get out of bed. And, after all, if these ads tell us we can be a Size 6 by New Year's Eve, we want desperately to believe them.

But here lies the problem. As vulnerable humans, we physically see ourselves as we are today. We mentally visualize an event in the future, like New Year's Eve, a class reunion, or a relative's wedding. We visualize ourselves thin and "perfect" at these future events. The ads for diet programs reinforce these visions with the dramatic "before" and "after" photos. But they fail to show us *the process* that must go on every day between present-day and future event.

If you've ever perused someone's photos of ongoing weight loss, taken once a week over a long period of time—say ten weeks-- you notice the progress is much less dramatic when viewed in small increments. That's the problem with setting long-term weight-loss goals. We stray and get lost during the lengthy journey because we can't really see the light at the end of the tunnel. We can imagine it, but we can't truly see it. And few of us have a faith that's strong enough to believe without seeing something that's actually within our short grasp.

Lesson eventually learned: "Keeping the faith" will help guide you to Heaven (and long-term weight loss). In the meantime, reinforce that faith by setting short-term, quickly attainable goals, like losing one or two pounds a week instead of losing 20 pounds in three months. That's a major key to Bucket List Weight Loss.

Another problem with the "Drop three pants sizes by New Year's" ads: We're led to believe that since it's so easy and such a sure thing, we might as well put it off until tomorrow or the following Monday. That gives us one last day of recreational overeating, which usually adds to another. Soon the New Year's Eve party is here, and we're the same size—or bigger—than we were when we first read about the "Drop three pants sizes" diet. It's almost as if weight-loss ads themselves are fattening!

Regardless, in 1978 I was duly inspired to give Stillman another try. I liked the extremely limited foods, and the fact that I could eat high protein (meat, eggs, cottage cheese) that truly satisfied my appetite and subdued my cravings after the first three hellish days of the diet. Quantities weren't limited; I liked that too. I could eat as much as I wanted of the allowed foods, without counting calories. Often I had nothing but diet sodas all day, and then went home to a dinner of cottage cheese and tuna mixed together. The pounds dropped off, and I went down two or three sizes within a few weeks.

There were just a couple problems. First, I was getting really sick of cottage cheese and tuna. Second, because I was bored with this type of eating, I was straying from the diet. The scale bounced up and down. One day I'd be "good" and stick with my Stillman plan, and the next morning I'd stop at Kroger on my way to work and pick up half a dozen pastries.

By this time, I was no longer working in the music business because I'd taken a full-time position with the Tennessee National Guard. I was required to wear an Army uniform to work every day, and to maintain a certain weight standard. Regulations on military weight and physical fitness tightened up. The periodic weigh-ins were just as humiliating as they had been in basic training. I truly didn't feel overweight, and thought I carried (in other words, hid) any excess poundage fairly well. Because I'd started a regular workout routine, I was in pretty good physical condition. But I was still haunted by the scale and the looming threat of discipline for exceeding the maximum allowable weight at the next weigh-in.

Lesson eventually learned: Make friends with your scale. Weighing yourself daily will help you handle the mental ups and downs of weight loss, and help you learn to accept yourself on a day-to-day basis. (More on "scale relationships" to follow....)

Exercise became even more important to me as a means of burning calories—especially on those days when I overindulged on pastries—but the exercise also increased my self esteem. I joined the YMCA and sometimes went there twice a day. I started jogging. I bought home exercise equipment. My social life dwindled because I spent so much time at the gym or working out at home. Sometimes I even conveniently forgot to eat, even though I'd make up for it the next day by stopping for another six pastries on my way to work. I could see the letters "OCD" (obsessive compulsive disorder) hovering over me, waiting to get stamped on my forehead. Binge eat, work out, binge eat, work out. You can get by with that lifestyle when you're in your 20s, but I began worrying about my future as I crowded 30.

1980. My weight was down to 172, but the military standards dictated I be closer to 165. That's when I discovered "Cambridge." More structure, but in a liquid form this time.

Meal replacement drinks had been around since the days of Jack LaLanne, but none had ever been marketed heavily and successfully until the Cambridge Diet. A can of Cambridge contained dry powder that, when mixed with water, turned into a fairly tasty shake. Cambridge was supposed to be very low in calories yet nutritionally complete. By "very low" we're talking 330 calories per day. It was supposed to simulate a starvation diet, while supplying all the basic nutrients needed to sustain life. If you wanted to crash weight off super-fast, you could drink Cambridge shakes (three a day, each 110 calories) and not die.

It was borderline insanity on my part, but I actually loved the stuff. It truly was satisfying to me, at least after the first three days when the hunger pains finally subsided. And I liked the fact that I didn't have to deal with, or even be around, "real" food. My downfall with eating real food was portion control. Once I started eating anything pleasurable, I found it difficult or impossible to stop until it was either gone or I felt icky. I enjoyed the sensation and the immediate gratification of food, and was typically so caught up in the moment that I blocked out any sense of future or consequence. One bite of pizza, ice cream, cookies or chips could cause me to literally eat like there was no tomorrow.

So Cambridge made it easy for me to simply avoid food altogether. I'd go on Cambridge alone for several days, watch five or six pounds drop off the scale, then start substituting my evening Cambridge with something I could chew and enjoy. That worked very well. In fact, I got down to 155 pounds for a few months and had to have my Army uniforms seriously altered. People were in awe of my success and I started hearing them say, "Now be careful not to lose too much." That was fun to hear, but I sensed a patronizing tone in their comments. Yes, I looked good...certainly better than when I weighed 190! But I still felt all-over "big." The weight loss had happened so quickly, my mind hadn't had time to adjust. I kept waiting to wake up from a dream and find myself back at 190 pounds.

Plus, I had these nagging fears:

1. Fear of food and of my inability to deal with real food and real eating. If I went to restaurants, to a friend's house for a dinner party, or to a social function, I'd have to go through the motions of eating like a normal person, all the while

resenting every morsel of solid food I was putting in my mouth, and fearing I'd "fall off the wagon" like a recovering alcoholic who slips.

2. Fear of running out of Cambridge. What if they stopped making the product? What if a nuclear attack destroyed the company? What if our national transportation system was shut down and no product could be shipped to dis-tributors? I was as psychologically dependent on this stuff as a druggy who needs her fix. I was hooked on fake food because I didn't think I could handle the real stuff anymore.

Yet the Cambridge Diet seemed to satisfy one very basic need for me: it offered me sufficient nutrition to keep my body going at near capacity while I lost weight. Maintaining my health and energy had become as important to me as dropping pounds. I was a compulsive exerciser, after all, and if I lost my health and energy, I wouldn't be able to exercise. That threat alone was enough to keep me from tipping the scales into anorexia. With the Cambridge drinks, I didn't experience low-blood-sugar shak-iness (even though I was consuming only 330 calories a day), and didn't feel like I was depleting my muscle tissue at all. Everything was good, until that day I almost killed myself at the Nashville YMCA.

Another annual weigh-in had been looming at work. I wanted to make sure I was well under the maximum allowed, which was at that time 168 pounds for a 5'10" female in my age group (I was 29.) The scheduled weigh-in was Friday. On Thursday I went all-out; I fasted, donated a pint of blood, and went to the Y, where I ran two miles and then took a sauna. After showering, I was sit-ting naked, a towel wrapped around me, on the bench in front of my locker when I realized I didn't have the strength to stand up and reach for my clothes. The world started going white. I knew I was passing out, so I leaned over and put my head between my legs. Some other women noticed my distress and came over to help. I was pale as ghost and clearly dehydrated. Someone brought me a small can of cold juice from the vending machine in the locker room. I believe the juice saved my life. I confessed to them what I'd done, but not why. Telling them about the upcoming military weigh-in was just too humiliating.

That incident was a wake-up call for me. Much as I wanted to be thin enough to pass my weigh-in, I wasn't willing to die for it. I didn't give up Cambridge entirely, but I didn't do anything quite as stupid as giving blood, fasting, and running two miles on the same day.

Lesson eventually learned: Bucket List Weight Loss is about becoming healthier by becoming thinner. If weight loss damages your health, you won't be able to enjoy the remainder of your life as a thin person.

Chapter 5

• • • • • •

A CHANGE OF
DIRECTION

In 1983 I voluntarily left my full-time National Guard job so I could revamp my life. I was an unattached Yankee female living in the Old South, and, while Nashville was still a fun place to live, I felt lonely and estranged from most of my peers who were married and raising kids. So I pulled up stakes and moved to Wyoming, where I planned to write a novel and find a rich, available rancher to marry.

I immediately bought a mountainside cabin, joined the YMCA, and fell in love. He was a rich rancher, but the romance ended badly, and I spent much of the first winter snowbound, eating Dinty Moore beef stew and drinking way too much alcohol. I got my exercise skiing, snowshoeing, hiking, and splitting firewood.

About that time my hip joints were both complaining rather loudly. The discomfort had started two years earlier in Nashville, but I'd chalked it up to "overuse injury" from too much time on a rowing machine. But by 1983 the pain and stiffness had dramatically increased. Excedrin got me through, since I had no health insurance.

In 1984 I met my future husband, who shared the same military background as I did, but lived in the state of Washington. By 1985 we were married and I moved to his dusty farm town on the "dry side" of the state. Except for my wonderful husband, there was nothing about the area I didn't loathe. It was a sprawling, flat-land town that suffered gray temperature inversions in the winter and dust storms in the hot summer.

In one fell swoop I'd given up my adventurous mountain life, the clean air of Wyoming, and my independence. But I'd finally found a good man. I was 32. It was time, I told myself, to grow up and learn to be a good wife.

My husband and I first lived in a small house on a crowded, busy, noisy street in town. Our house felt like a fish bowl. I got a part-time job as a weight-training instructor at the local YMCA, and sold a few magazine articles. But aside from that, I felt like a fish out of water. Resentment welled up in me. I silently refused to assimilate into the agricultural community. I ached for Wyoming and all that I'd left behind. When hubby went across the state for weekend National Guard drills, I'd burrow in at home with a stack of rented chick flicks, a couple half-gallons of ice cream, and a box of deli chicken. That was my fun and comfort.

Lesson eventually learned: Depression eating creates more depression. If you eat because you feel bad, you'll still feel bad after you ate and you'll feel even worse when you step back on the scale. However, if you fight the urge to eat when you're depressed, you may still be depressed the next day....but you'll be thinner! It's a whole lot more pleasant to be depressed and thin than depressed and fat.

The hip pain and stiffness were getting worse, and I self-pre-scribed more exercise in a resolve to keep strong and limber. Frankly I was afraid to stop exercising, for fear I'd seize up like the Tin Man. I figured exercise was the best thing to keep the joints loose. Plus, the endorphins released during a workout gave my sagging spirits a physiological boost. My weight yo-yoed twenty pounds several times over the next few years, and my clothing ran from a Size 10 to a Size 14. I refused to buy any Size 16; that became my self-imposed ceiling. If the 14s got tight, I'd take drastic steps then and there.

Shopping for a Size 14 isn't particularly fun. Or shopping for any size that accommodates a 40-pound weight excess. Even if you can find clothing that fits over your fat rolls, it just doesn't look the way it's supposed to. It's not what the designer envisioned for her garments! Straining in the hips, tight or gaping in the waist, bulges on the thighs, pockets that pucker...shopping is much harder when you're large, because you have to try on three times as many things in order to find something that's passable.

Shopping this way is also expensive, because once you finally find a pair of pants that fit, you buy five pairs. Larger clothes usually cost more too.

Lesson eventually learned: When you get to be a small size, shopping becomes easy, fun and affordable! You'll find stuff in discount stores and even thrift shops that looks fantastic and feels comfortable on you. The irony: you won't need as exten-sive a wardrobe when you're thin, because anything will look good on you. It's the body people will notice, not the paper sack you're wearing!

The hip pain continued to worsen, and I sought medical advice when my husband was finally able to add me to his employees' health insurance plan. I saw half a dozen doctors and specialists in the next couple years, and no one diagnosed or effectively treated the problem. A healthy, active female, 35 years old, with bilateral hip pain? It had to be muscle strain, or a femoral hernia, or spinal misalignment, or..... The docs were all looking for something unusual—certainly not plain old arthritis.

Eventually I got a definitive diagnosis from someone who actually knew how to read x-rays. It was plain old osteoarthritis. This is the "wear and tear" kind of arthritis that affects nearly everyone over the age of 60 to some degree. At age 40, I'd already worn mine out through repetitive exercise, coupled with a genetic predisposition. (Both my brother and sister eventually had major joint replacements too.) The prognosis: I needed bilateral hip replacements.

In January 1993, I had my left hip replaced. With the new joint parts, I was immediately free of the pain that had nagged me for ten years. Now that I was reclaiming my youth, I couldn't wait to start a new exercise routine and get my weight down once again. My recovery was quick. Within five weeks I was riding my horse again.

One year later I had my right hip replaced. Total hip replacements are miraculous surgeries, able to instantly alleviate joint pain and allow people to have nearly full use of their hip joints again. The only down side—and it's pretty small in relation to the up side—is the disfigurement aspect. You don't hear much about that, again probably because it's just not that important in the grand scheme of things. Nonetheless, hip replacements can really mess up the figures of mature women who already have normal saddlebags on their thighs. The problem is with the incision. A surgeon will slice open the saddlebag to access the joint, and then attempt to sew it back up when the surgery is complete. Since fat pads tend to shift with gravity, it's difficult for a surgeon to realign everything and sew it up just as it was. Many patients end up with saddlebags that weren't exactly where they used to be. The displaced fat seems trapped around the long incision, like a new appendage.

The "new" saddlebags totally changed my shape and the way my clothes fit. Finding pants and jeans that would accommodate— and hide--my fat pillows was difficult, and I resigned myself to never wearing conventional bathing suits or stretchy pants again.

Physical deformities aside, I enjoyed a new lease on life with two new, virtually pain-free hips. I hiked, cross-country skied, rode horses, started a new dog-training business that kept me hopping 12 hours a day, and exercised daily on my home equipment: the Nordic Trak, a Schwinn Air-Dyne stationary bike, an eliptical trainer, and a mini-trampoline. The hips lasted through eight good years of this gleeful abuse, and then started hinting to me that their usefulness was over. Pain and stiffness returned. I'd worn them out.

Lesson eventually learned: You need joint replacements? Get them! Don't let the doctors discourage you by saying you're "too young." Reclaim your life and live it to the fullest, pain-free. Just don't expect hip replacements to last forever if you're fairly young and active. They're a bit like brake pads on cars. They wear out if you use them a lot, and you may be back in the shop getting a second set installed within five to fifteen years...

2002. It was a hot August, and my weight was back up in the 180s. The hips, now eight and nine years old, hurt like hell. I lived on "Vitamin E" (Excedrin) and had only made the hip pain worse by trying to exercise away the excess weight.

I'd heard about Weight Watchers, although my loyalty was still with Stillman and Cambridge. But when my best friend Laurie told me about the Weight Watchers program she'd just started, my ears perked up. Laurie had about 80 pounds to lose and had lost seven in the first week. She wasn't hungry either.

She explained the Weight Watchers "points" system, and how daily menu planning became almost game-like. She was eating a great variety of foods, with basically no restrictions on many vegetables and fruits. She was purchasing lots of low-fat versions of normally high-fat foods (cheese, yogurt, milk), which allowed her to eat large quantities and still stay within the program limits. She was also going to Weight Watchers meetings. I told her the program sounded good, but not the meetings. I had neither time nor interest in support groups. Her recommendation: try the on-line version. Two hours later I was sitting at my computer, signed up and perusing the Weight Watchers website.

Like many others, I embraced Weight Watchers with a passion and dropped about five pounds the first week. The on-line version was perfect for me because it demanded accountability while providing anonymity. From Weight Watchers I learned to control my portions, keep track of my caloric intake, lower my fat consumption, and eat more vegetables. The food choices were endless, because Weight Watchers doesn't limit what you can have. If you choose to have a high-calorie dessert, you just make up for it by eating less of other things. You're assigned an allowable number of "points" you can eat per day, based on your weight. When I began the program, my weight bracket called for 24 to 28 points a day. Figuring that one Weight Watchers "point" roughly equals 50 calories, and that most green vegetables have no point value at all, it's easy to see how a person can stay full—and healthy—following the Weight Watchers plan.

I became a Weight Watchers fiend for the next few months, as I saw the weight melt away, seemingly with little or no effort or hunger. In November of that year, I celebrated my 50th birthday and felt smashingly beautiful in a size 8.

But Weight Watchers posed a couple unexpected problems for me. The program requires you to "journal" everything you eat and drink, which is normally a great habit. Each evening I'd sit down in front of the website and do my points calculations for the day. Did I "eat enough points?" Did I meet the dairy requirements? How much fiber had I eaten? Did I drink enough water? Did I record my exercise points?

Talk about a trigger for an obsessive/compulsive person! While Weight Watchers is an excellent program, I started to feel I was a slave to it. The game of "How much can I eat and stay within the limits?" ceased being fun because it began to rule my life. Now I was thinking about food more than ever, and that led to cravings. Especially for cookies.

With Weight Watchers, you can eat anything you want—even cookies--in moderation. But that was my problem. I'd drive to the supermarket and buy a dozen bakery cookies with the intention of eating just one or two and giving the rest to my husband. By the time I got home, most of the cookies were gone, so I'd leave the cookie bag in the car and polish off the remainder the next day while driving to work.

So even with Weight Watchers' indisputably wonderful program, I failed when it came to cravings and portion control. It was so much like being a drug addict or an alcoholic. If I could totally avoid the temptations by not having cookies, chips or delectable leftovers calling my name, then I could stay "food-sober." That's why the super-restrictive diets like Stillman and Cambridge had appealed to me. But I knew I couldn't live the rest of my life on programs like those. *I wanted more control than that. I wanted to be freed of the burden.* Okay...I wanted to have my cake and eat it too.

Recovering substance abusers deserve tons of respect. They're surrounded by society's temptations and have to constantly keep up their guard. "Food addicts" have an even harder time, since we all need food for sustenance. We can't eliminate food from our lives, like alcohol or drugs. The fact that we're deluged with food ads on radio, TV and billboards doesn't help, nor does the fact that obesity has become socially acceptable.

Lesson eventually learned: Your biggest challenge in weight loss may not be you, but rather the people who surround you. This is the time to start prioritizing and putting yourself (your health and well being) first. Visualize yourself strong, lean and confident, and standing on a pedestal above those who are trying to push food at you. Let them push it at each other instead. Stand tall and become a role model for them. That may be the greatest gift you can give them.

Besides cravings, portion control and recordkeeping, my other HUGE problem with Weight Watchers was--um--gas. Okay, folks, I'm not talking a little gas that can be moderated with Beano. I'm talking major, chronic, painful, bloating, and pesky gas that sometimes simply couldn't be held back. That's what beans, most vegetables, and high-fiber bread did to me. There were so many wonderful "good-for-me" foods that I could eat in abundance on the Weight Watchers plan, but my body couldn't handle them.

"Give it time," the experts say. "Adjust slowly. Drink lots of water. Your body will learn to process the fiber."

It didn't happen. Ever. At the time, I owned a dog-training business that had me teaching group classes six days a week. It was impossible for me to do my job—running over to this student, dashing back over to another, chasing dogs around the room, or jumping up and down to make a point—if I was constantly worried about my own "barking."

Reluctantly, I gave up on Weight Watchers. I was forlorn; arguably the best diet program in the world hadn't worked for me, and I had no idea where to turn next. I simply couldn't live with the pain and discomfort caused by good foods like yogurt, oatmeal, whole grain breads, and most fruits and vegetables. The 25 pounds I'd dropped on the program came back in a matter of months.

2003: Atkins
My friend Laurie is another yo-yo dieter. She'd long since abandoned Weight Watchers for reasons of her own, and was now doing the Atkins low-carb diet, again with pretty good success.

As she explained it to me, it sounded a lot like my old favorite Stillman, but with more than just meat, eggs and water. Stillman had been for short-term use, was exceptionally hard on the kidneys, and was very restrictive. The Atkins diet was much more liberal, seemed to be more healthful and rounded, and was touted as a lifetime way of eating. Best of all, I wouldn't have to eat all those gas-inducing breads and vegetables.

Discovering Atkins was like reuniting with an old friend who had matured. The high-fat, high-protein, low-carbohydrate combination was delightful. Granted, the first three to five days of "induction" were rough, as my system weaned itself of extra carbs and sugar. But I knew the headaches, shakes and queasiness were temporary, like a hangover, and that I'd feel much better once I'd weathered that storm. The weight came off at a fairly steady, predictable rate. Best of all, cravings disappeared. Any time I felt like I was denying myself, I could microwave a delicious chicken breast or cook up a couple hamburger patties. The fat and protein does a much better job of satisfying my body—and the mind—than a can of green beans or even a bag of potato chips.

The Atkins diet was exceedingly popular at the time. I knew several people who'd done Atkins and lost tremendous amounts of weight. But nearly every person gained back the weight—plus some extra—as soon as they went off Atkins. It was ridiculously predictable.

"I don't want to be like that," I resolved. The only way to avoid the rebound was to make Atkins a way of life, and I planned to do that. For nearly four years I stayed faithful to Dr. Atkins' plan. I was back down to a stable size 8 and felt terrific. I subsisted pretty much on meat and salad, and had planned to live the rest of my life that way.

2005. A trip to Hawaii messed up my plans.
Lesson eventually learned: Never say "Never" about anything. Life--and eating regimens--really must be taken one day at a time.

My two all-time favorite foods are chicken and fresh pineapple. The chicken is quite compatible with Atkins, but pineapple is

48

not—at least, not in the quantities I wanted to consume during that Hawaiian vacation with four other women. Our first stop after getting off the plane in Maui was Costco. We loaded up gondolas full of fresh pineapple, croissants, coconut shrimp, Macadamian nuts, cheeses, wine, obligatory salad greens and, yes, rotisserie chicken. I'd decided to cave in and eat as much fresh pineapple as I wanted during this trip. It was Paradise, after all.

Guess what! We all ate and drank in excess and had a blast doing it. By the last day of our trip I was polishing up the last of the buttery croissants! I knew it would be difficult to go back on Atkins and re-cleanse my system once I left Hawaii. I loved Atkins, but the divine pleasure of eating fresh fruit made me question whether or not I really wanted to restrict myself to meat and green salads for the rest of my life.

That little seed of doubt was the only excuse I needed to abandon Atkins for good.

2007. A banner year. My husband and I retired from our businesses and left Washington. Three years earlier we'd purchased 40 beautiful acres in northwest Montana and had begun construction on our retirement dream home. I envisioned myself in a beautiful new kitchen, cooking up delectable crockpot meals that would allow me to play outside all day and come in at night to fragrant, home-cooked dinners. With lots of carbohydrates.

The house wasn't finished when we finally arrived in Montana on Dec. 1, 2007, so we spent three months of Montana winter in a 5th wheel trailer with our three large, hairy dogs. It was a great adventure, but we went basically all winter without looking in a full-length mirror. We wore bulky clothing to keep warm. We slept ten hours a night. During the days, we amused ourselves by playing cards, reading, and eating. Needless to say, by the time we moved into our beautiful home that spring, we were both filling out our bulky clothing pretty well. Hubby had gained about 15 pounds, and I'd swelled back up to 185+. I worried that, once I got all my clothing unpacked in the new house, I wouldn't be able to fit into any of them. I wasn't off base by much.

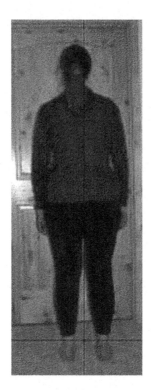

Chapter 6

• • • • • •

LIFE IN DENIAL

Big and happy

We live in one of the most beautiful yet economically depressed parts of the country. Our neighbors are either hard-working ranchers or loggers, or they're retired people who migrated to this neck of the woods because they like the simple, quiet, down-to-earth lifestyle. They love the outdoors and solitude. They're not the least bit pretentious. Most are not too concerned about being ten, twenty, or even fifty pounds overweight. Typically they gain a few pounds during the long, dark, inactive winter months and lose it again in the spring when they begin gardening, fishing, hiking, and splitting wood for the next winter.

So it was easy to resign myself to the idea of being Big For Life. My Size 8s either went to the guest room closet or I gave them away. I did keep a pair of Size 6 L.L. Bean jeans I'd bought and worn (for about three weeks) five years earlier. For some reason I couldn't bear to part with them. Even back when they fit, they'd been snug. But I'd gotten them on and zipped, and I never wanted to forget that I once wore a size 6, even if it was only until I ate a large meal.

I decided to never diet again. It was time to accept the way I was, and to enjoy life to the fullest. The diets hadn't worked, I'd always gained the weight back, and I no longer wanted to live with such regimentation in my life. Besides, it didn't really matter anymore how I looked. I wasn't trying to impress anyone.

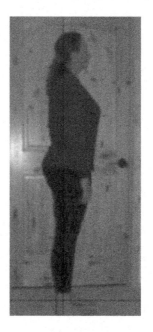

Big and hurting

It's funny how we can talk ourselves into accepting just about anything. You're fat? No, you're not, you're just big-boned! You don't like to exercise? Well, you get enough exercise walking up and down the stairs in your house. Now you're buying Size 18 pants? Well, they cut these garments so small and tight these days...

Having spent a winter without looking in mirrors and several sub-sequent years without stepping on a scale earned me Resident Status In The State of Denial. I was chubby, dumb and happy in retirement life. I enjoyed my physical activities—hiking, horse-back riding, lake kayaking, and dog agility—as best I could, and took pride in the fact that I could indeed do those things quite capably at the age of 57. But I was continually suffering setbacks in my training. I could work out on a treadmill for 35 minutes, but not for 45 without suffering aches the next day. I could paddle my kayak for two hours without fatigue, but the next day an elbow would be screaming "Lay off me!"

My big body was setting limits I considered unreasonable. In retaliation I'd take a couple Excedrin around mid-day. It's always been my "drug of choice," much more effective for me than any other NSAID. But the Excedrin actually perpetuated the problem; I'd feel so much better after taking it that I'd immediately go out and overdo again. It was a vicious cycle.

I chalked most of it up to the aging process, mostly because people all around me were doing the same thing. The laments of the over-50 population are numerous.

"I can hardly get out of bed in the morning anymore."

"Everything hurts these days."

"It's only going to get worse."

"Getting old is the pits."

"I just can't do 'that' anymore."

You actually hear more "younger" seniors complaining than the older ones, as if it's a badge of honor to be joining the "Perpetually in Pain" club. Frankly I think it's an excuse for a lot of folks that age to just give up. If everyone else in your social group is bemoaning the aches and pains of aging, it's a lot easier for you to throw in the towel and jump into the pity party. If you're surrounded by friends who no longer seem to care about their looks, their weight, fitness level or overall health, it's tempting to join in the apathy.

In fact, if you decide *not* to sink into the apathetic abyss with your peers—if you make a true effort to maintain or improve your weight, fitness and health—you may even be scrutinized by those you leave behind in the mire. I have a sister who's eight years older than I am. She has severe health problems, largely caused or aggravated by lifestyle choices she's made. A while back she asked me not to share my successes—basically, my weight loss, health, activities, competitive achievements and overall personal happiness and satisfaction—with her anymore. In other words, she didn't want to hear about my great new life. She wasn't interested in sharing my joy; she only felt bitter and resentful.

You may lose some friends too, as you start to realize your *Bucket List Weight Loss.* They may feel threatened by your success and happiness. They will find fault with how you achieved your goal. They will criticize you for doing it. Be prepared. Not everyone loves winners.

On the other hand, you're going to influence and inspire a great many more people—some you haven't even met yet—to improve their health and happiness, to continue living and learning, and to start enjoying a life they'd dared only dream about.

Getting fat and lazy would have been very easy at age 57 when I was retired, living a life of relative leisure, and no longer trying to impress anyone in business or social circles. But if I succumbed to becoming fat and lazy, I'd have to forego the activities I loved the most--the same activities that made me feel like a kid. Playing outside, being physical, pushing myself to that wonderful

feeling of exhaustion that tells me my body parts are still functioning and capable, despite the aging process....those are the
activities that invigorate and revive me. They're the activities that
make me feel youthful rather than geriatric. I didn't want to give
them up. After all, I lived in a virtual paradise for the outdoor-
lover, with endless trails to hike and ride, and countless lakes and
streams to explore.

I trained for a half-marathon in 2010 and completed the whole
13.1 miles successfully at a fast walk. I would have run some of it,
but it hurt too much. I wrote it off to "bad hips and knees," but if
I'd stepped on a scale I would have been slapped in the face with
the real reason: 30 pounds of excess weight bouncing around
on those poor joints. I avoided scales like the plague and lived
in a fantasy world of denial. How could I possibly have a weight
problem? I'd just completed a half-marathon!

*Lesson eventually learned: We can fool ourselves into thinking
that weight really doesn't matter--that it's more important to be
strong and healthy. But excess weight on joints is a deal killer.
Whether it's five pounds of retained water or five pounds of extra fat, it's a five-pound burden for which our joints were not
designed! Weight DOES matter!*

Chapter 7

• • • • • •

THE GREAT
FOOD REVOLT

Now that I wasn't following a specific diet regimen, I was eating the same foods I prepared for my husband--meat, potatoes, veggies, salads, breads, and occasional desserts. I was getting pretty irritated at my chronically irritated bowels. It was hard to believe that wholesome foods like bananas, peanut butter, oatmeal and granola could be bad for me, but there was no denying it; four hours after eating any of those things, I was feeling miserable and lethargic with intestinal gas, bloating, and sometimes headaches.

So I started making a list of the foods that made me feel "bad."

- Bananas and banana bread.

- Oatmeal.

- Potatoes.

- Pasta.

- Various nuts.

- Dairy products.

- Bread.

- Granola.

- Oranges.

- Tomatoes.

- Onions.

What was the correlation between these wholesome foods? What was it that made my gut react with such venom? Was it really the individual foods, the combination of foods, or was it just all coincidence?

In November of 2010, I had lunch at a local eatery with a bunch of neighbor women. I ordered some kind of sandwich with french fries. Big, crisp, greasy, golden, gorgeous fries. I ate them all. Four hours later my stomach was doing somersaults and my intestines were protesting the onslaught of heavy food cooked in old grease. It took several hours for things to work their way through my system. During that time I contemplated those fries. They'd looked good, and the first couple tasted fine. I can't really remember how the rest tasted, because I was eating mindlessly and paying more attention to the conversations going on around me. I was eating because the food was sitting in front of me, because I paid for it, and because my friends were doing the same thing. But in retrospect, as I sat at home feeling my stomach gurgle, those fries hadn't been good enough to make this agony worthwhile.

Lesson eventually learned: Social time is about socializing, not about eating. If you're out with friends, make due with a salad or a glass of iced tea. If your friend's plate looks more inviting than yours, remember she will suffer the consequences of eating all that stuff. You, on the other hand, will be thinner, healthier, and happier...and you still will have enjoyed a good visit over lunch!

That was basically the last time I ate potatoes in any quantity. It was easy to give them up. All I had to say to myself was this: "They're not worth it." I've since noticed that potato chips have the same effect on me. Again, I tell myself, "They're not worth it." With this in mind, it's easy to turn them down.

Potatoes are such a part of mainstream America's diet that I knew I'd have to find a substitute if I was never going to have another bake potato in a restaurant.

That's how I discovered brown rice. Until then, all rice in my life had been white. Brown rice was for ex-hippies, liberals, and vegetarians who only bought organic foods and did yoga sun salutations every morning. Then at age 58, I cooked up a batch of brown rice for the first time in my life. I ate it plain, with no adornment, not even salt. It was out of this world!! Much to my utter amazement, the brown rice had taste, texture, and visual appeal. It required chewing, it had a wonderful nuttiness, and it was extremely filling and satisfying. Not only that, but I learned brown rice was an excellent source of protein. Fiber content was high too, and that part frankly worried me. I half expected to blow up like a hot-air balloon in about four hours.

But the hours passed. My gut remained quiet; my energy level was good! I felt a mild, healthy hunger by evening, but I had no great craving to overeat that night. Brown rice, it seemed, got along very well with my body.

So I started thinking about the other starchy carbohydrate that wreaked havoc with my system: bread. Not just white bread, either. In fact, the worst offenders were the healthful whole-grain breads. Much as I loved bread's taste, texture and aroma, I knew that if I ate them, I'd have severe gastric distress in four hours. Eating bread wasn't worth the discomfort. Besides, the brown rice could also substitute for the bread. With brown rice I'd be getting my easy-to-digest carbohydrates, which would keep me fueled and energized for a busy, active day. Plus, I'd be getting protein. As long as I didn't overdo it by eating too much, brown rice appeared to be my saving grace.

I began experimenting with various additives that would add new flavor dimensions to the brown rice: Parmesan cheese, spinach, pineapple, Italian seasoning, lean meats left over from the previous night's dinner. I ate it hot and cold. It was great as a warm breakfast cereal with soy milk and a little sweetener. It was the perfect quick snack if I needed an energy boost. Best of all, it was kind to my digestive system.

Until that point I'd heard of gluten intolerances and Celiac disease, but I never truly thought I was afflicted. Sometimes it seemed EVERYTHING gave me gas—not just wheat products--and other times I'd be gas-free for several days in a row. Was there something missing in my gut? Did I need probiotics? Why did good foods like oatmeal and bananas do a number on me? Did I actually have serious food intolerances? Food allergies?

I didn't have the time or resources to go through an extensive battery of allergy testing. So I decided to simply stop eating foods that were upsetting my body. The list grew to include potatoes in any form, products made with potato flour, dairy in any form except small quantities of hard cheeses (like Parmesan), sweet potatoes, oatmeal, barley, wheat in any form, citrus fruit, apples, bananas, tomatoes and tomato products, pea soup, peanuts, almonds, and peanut butter. I knew I'd still get gas from beans, broccoli, cabbage, brussel sprouts and cauliflower. That was a given. But if I mixed them in very small quantities with brown rice, the results were tolerable.

Lesson eventually learned: Listen to your body. Get to know how it feels about certain foods going through its system. If it tells you it can't handle x-food very well, respect it enough to not feed it x-food. Your body knows best what it needs, but you have to listen to it!

A few weeks into my personally designed "elimination diet," a couple interesting things started happening.

1. My appetite decreased. My system was satisfied with less food.

2. Cravings for carbohydrates—sweets, breads, even alcohol—disappeared.

Holy moley!! Not only had I eliminated my chronic gas problem, but I'd found a way to stop the cravings and eat less!

It was almost too good to believe, so I remained a skeptic.. How much of these results were physical? How much were psychological? I have no idea, but I do know the two work in consort. Suddenly I was consuming way fewer calories and—even more noteworthy—I was spending lots less time THINKING about food. My energy level was high, because my body wasn't wasting energy dealing with gastric discomfort. So I was moving more and burning more calories. My clothes were getting looser! I assumed I was losing weight too, but dared not step on a scale to face the truth.

Chapter 8

• • • • • •

HELLO, SCALE!

No one loves scales. Like many people, I avoid them whenever possible.

The aversion to scales started when I was in grade school. Twice a year we'd march as a class to the nurse's office for height/weight checks. I didn't understand at the time how those little sliding weight things worked, or how to read the scale, but I knew some kids definitely made the scale go "Clank!" more easily than others, and I still recall kids in line giggling when a hefty kid stepped on the scale. I remember being one of those bigger kids, since I was the tallest girl in my class. And I remember my mom counseling me at home later when she heard how much weight I'd gained since the last weigh-in. Even then, she was instilling her own weight consciousness in me.

The scale had been a nemesis during my Army career too. When that was over, I still had to step on a damn scale every time I saw a doctor. I learned to look away and not read the weight when I stood on it. I'm sure the nurses weighing me couldn't have cared less; they weren't going to gasp in horror at the number on the scale, so why should I? My weight was whatever it was, and I didn't need to know. I didn't want to know either, because ignorance is of course bliss...and denial. If I don't know what I weigh,

I don't have to deal with it. I can live in a fantasy world, thinking I'm ten pounds lighter than I actually am.

There's always been a conventional bathroom scale in our house. The current one (hiding in the basement) is the old-fashioned spring kind with a needle that bounces around unless you stand perfectly still. If you put more weight on the balls of your feet, it reads a pound lighter than if you're standing on your heels. How do you trust a scale like that! I won't set foot on it anymore. When we first got it, I could climb on it three times in a row and get three progressively heavier results. So I'd fiddle with the little adjustment wheel on it, but then it would weigh too light. I shoved it into a corner in the basement because I couldn't handle what it did to my self esteem every time I got on it.

During the Atkins years, I avoided the scale because all the literature said I should pay attention to the fit of my clothes instead. Atkinsites believe that if you get on the scale and aren't pleased with the results, you'll go off the diet in frustration. So I only snuck onto the scale a handful of times in four years…and, sure enough, I was fairly disappointed every time I did. The weight loss was never what I thought it should be. The clothes were looser, but the progress was so slow! They say that the weight doesn't matter? Well, it mattered to me. That's why I quit weighing myself altogether for the next several years.

Living without weighing, however, can set you into a horrible downward spiral. If you never really know for sure what your weight is, you don't worry so much about a few days of overeating. Pretty soon "a few days" becomes more days than you can remember, overeating becomes the norm, and suddenly you become suspicious that your clothes are shrinking in the dryer.

In March of 2010, I finally made peace with a scale and forever changed my relationship with it. This became the single biggest factor in my *Bucket List Weight Loss*.

My neighbor, Lorraine, invited me over to see the Nintendo Wii Fit game she'd gotten for Christmas from her kids. I'd heard about the Wii, but didn't really understand how it worked. She told me about the exercise programs it offfered. The games you could play on it. The record-keeping feature that tracked your weight and fitness. The interactive personal trainer who coached you through a workout.

I'd read reviews about the Wii Fit program. People said it was truly like having a personal trainer...and a lot less expensive! Even with a basement full of exercise equipment, I still thought it would be fun to have that "personal trainer" thing going on. And the games sounded fun.

She let me try it. I stepped on the Wii Fit Balance Board sitting on the floor in front of their TV screen, followed the commands, and created my own personal "Mii"--a cartoonish figure that looked sort of like me and actually represented me on the screen. The Balance Board weighed me and told me my bodyfat percentage based on my height, weight and age. The animated voice was friendly and completely nonjudgmental. The Balance Board also checked my core stability, and then ran me through a couple exercises to check my center of gravity and basic balance abilities. It was fun! The friendly, instant feedback was great! So were the little fitness tips that were interjected in between the exercises. I loved this thing!!

Next we tried a couple of the interactive exercise programs. You could choose from yoga, strength training, aerobics, and balance games, each offering lots of variety, instant feedback, and gratification. It even kept track of how many minutes you were "working out." Before I knew it, I'd been active on the Wii Fit Balance Board for 30 minutes, and was just getting warmed up!

Lorraine also let me try the Wii Sports DVD, which included interactive tennis, golf, baseball and bowling. Playing tennis with this TV was more fun than I'd had in a long time. Best of all, I was getting a moderate workout while playing. I actually felt like Chrissie Evert! (For any youngsters reading this, Chris was the World No. 1 Singles tennis player throughout the 1970s and early 1980s.)

I went home and ordered the Nintendo Wii console, the Wii Fit software, and the Wii Fit Balance Board off the internet. I couldn't wait to get started on my own program, but little did I suspect the impact it would have on my life.

It arrived the next week in a couple small boxes, and took me about 15 minutes to set it up. I'd worried about that, because I'm a disaster with power cords, instructions in fine print, and anything that has to do with programming. But the Wii Fit stuff went together like huge jigsaw puzzle pieces, and in minutes I was ready to try it out.

What a great concept, this Wii Fit program! It makes exercise fun. It challenges you to compete against yourself. It's motivating. It's cute and friendly. It charts your progress, gently counsels you if you backslide, and even remembers your birthday. EVEN THE WEIGH-IN is bearable. There's something about having an interactive high-tech digital gizmo weighing me that makes me trust its totally objective accuracy. Particularly when it then advises me (very politely) of my "ideal weight" and how much I have to lose to get there. It really is like having a personal trainer, a secret coach with whom you can share that awful secret of how much you weigh.

Since we got it, the Wii Fit program has changed our lives. My husband and I both weigh every morning and take the little balance tests to determine our "virtual age." He's usually around 30 years old, and I'm typically 42. Considering our actual ages are decades older, it's an upbeat way to start the day.

The built-in Balance Board scale got me comfortable facing my own weight each and every morning. When it showed a drop of one pound after the first day, I was hooked. By seeing the weight presented that way--in numbers and in several graphs, and with vocal encouragement from the animated character on the screen--I could accept the findings as trustworthy and objective. At last I had a starting point: 183.6 pounds. It was what it was. The Wii Fit program had sparked a little fire of personal competition within myself. Tomorrow, I thought, if I make some minor changes in what I eat and drink today, and in how much I exercise, just maybe I can be down to 182 and see that on the graph.

It worked. I was on my way.

Chapter 9

• • • • • •

HOW I DID IT

What you've read so far tells you how I got to this point in my weight-watching life. Everything we experience teaches us a lesson. If we're lucky, we get to put all the lessons together and make them work for us once we mature. Being over 50 is just wonderful, because you finally have the wisdom and experiences to make the remainder of your life as pleasurable and productive as possible. It's even more wonderful if your health is good and you're not carrying any excess weight.

As I began my *Bucket List Weight Loss* journey in April 2011, weighing in at 183.6 pounds, I started writing down the changes I was making in my eating and lifestyle habits. *None of these changes had been done with losing weight in mind.* They'd come about because I wanted to feel better and move better for the rest of my life. It just so happened that the weight started melting off me as I applied them.

Bucket List Weight Loss consists of 11 concepts or habits. They all work in consort to give you a more comfortable life with a great side benefit: you automatically lose all the weight you want to lose.

With these 11 concepts etched in my brain, I know I won't gain back the weight I've lost. Can you understand how wonderful that is? I know I'll be able to maintain my Size 4-6 for at least the remainder of my active years. All the energy I'd wasted obsessing over food and my bigness has been freed up to use on much more productive things. The excess weight is gone for good. That's because *Bucket List Weight Loss* is not a diet; it's a way of living. It's not something you "do" to lose weight and then stop doing. Again, it really has little to do with losing weight. That's just one of the happy results.

It's not dieting we're talking about. **It's living!**

One more word before we get into "the list." This is MY list. It's worked a miracle for me, and I'm sharing it with you. That doesn't mean you have to eat brown rice just because I do. That doesn't mean you have to give up oatmeal or bananas just because I do. Part of the beauty of *Bucket List Weight Loss* is that you personalize it and make it work for you. My list is food for your thoughts. May it help your Bucket List dream come true.

The 11 Steps
to
Bucket List Weight Loss

BLWL Concept 1: "Four hours from now"
Think four hours ahead before you eat that.
How will your gut feel? How will your mind and joints feel? Do
you want to avoid being gassy? Remember the HANGOVER
syndrome.

The original reason I started this whole *BLWL* lifestyle change was to eliminate gas and indigestion. I wasn't thinking about losing weight. That's why "Think four hours ahead" is at the top of the list.

What will you be doing four hours from right now? Where will you be? Going out for dinner? Giving a lecture? Sitting on the sideline at the soccer field? Making love?

And how would you like to feel when you're there? Gassy, bloated, stiff, and inflamed? Unable to move because you're holding back flatulence? Or thin and lithe, able to suck in your gut and move easily and gracefully, without pain?

As chronic dieters, most of us have enough trouble seeing past the present moment if a favorite food temptation is staring us in the face. "Lose two pants sizes in six weeks" sounds good in an ad, but we tend to forget that six weeks is 42 days of difficult self discipline. That's 1,008 hours of eating abnormally and denying ourselves the foods we love most.

But if you think *just four hours ahead*—which is about how long it takes for food to start digesting and working its way into your colon—you can plan for intestinal comfort when you need it most.

Once again, I hearken back to my dog-training classes. I loved to gulp down those bakery cookies on my way to work, and my favorites were the Costco oatmeal/raisin cookies. I didn't realize it then, but the combination of wheat flour, oatmeal, and raisins was just about lethal to my gut. Four hours after eating them, a gas attack would catch up to me in the middle of a dog-training demonstration with 20 people sitting in front of me. Most of the time I could hold it in, but there were a few occasions when a "bark" sneaked out. Oh, I'd talk faster and louder then, hoping everyone was so engrossed in my demo that they didn't hear. But I always wondered about the conversations on their drives home from class. "Did you hear her fart?" "Was that what it was? I thought it was that dog's butt hitting the floor when it sat..."

As if that wasn't bad enough, I'd often polish off a few more cookies on my way home at 8 p.m. That was a timing problem too. Four hours later I'd be saying something like, "Not tonight, honey, I have bad gas."

With you, it may not be a gas issue. It could be a mobility issue, or simply a self esteem issue. Eating foods that your body doesn't readily accept or digest can make you feel lethargic, bloated, headachy, or just achy everywhere else. In other words, it can make you feel lousy. Eating too much can do the same thing.

You will suffer, just as predictably as you will suffer from a hangover if you drink too much. Time will heal you, of course. But who wants to *ever* feel that horrible? Are six margaritas really worth suffering nausea, headache, chills and dizziness for 24 hours? Of course not! After you've experienced a hangover once or twice, you learn to limit yourself because the consequences are too unpleasant if you don't.

Why not look at food the same way? Once you start realizing which foods give you a "hangover" four hours later, you'll find it easy to avoid them. In fact, you won't want anything to do with them. Potato chips used to be a huge temptation for me until I discovered they were so gas-producing that I was miserable after I ate them. Remembering that, I now have absolutely no desire for them. Same thing with ice cream, and many other former temptations. I recall how lousy I feel after I eat them, and it becomes an easy choice to leave them alone.

Think of the last time you overindulged in foods you knew weren't good for you, or foods that made you feel bloated or lethargic. They were probably wheat-based, sugary, greasy or dairy. If you choose not to have a hangover from one of these groups, simply avoid them...or exercise extreme moderation, just as you would with any alcoholic drinks known to knock you for a loop.

Nearly all of us have food sensitivities of one kind or another these days. I didn't have mine diagnosed by a medical professional, because I discovered my own ways of dealing with them: mainly, avoiding the foods that caused them. Do I have Celiac Disease? Probably not. But that doesn't mean my body likes gluten products; it clearly doesn't. By avoiding them, as well as avoiding dairy (yes, I am lactose intolerant) and the other foods on my verboten list, I'm also avoiding the unpleasant reactions.

Feeling good, physically and mentally, is really what my program is all about. Feeling good for two minutes (during and immediately after you've ingested something yummy but deadly) isn't what I'm talking about. You need to feel good several hours later. If you know you will feel worse in four hours, avoid eating that particular food.

Homework: Write down the foods that you know definitely "don't agree" with you, along with the ones you suspect. Find correlations between the foods. Dairy? High fiber cereal? Bread?? Next, write down the symptoms you feel several hours after eating each of the "disagreeable" foods. Finally, imagine yourself eliminating those pain-causing foods from your diet and never feeling those upsetting symptoms again!

BLWL Concept 2: "Gut talk"
Ask your body what it wants to eat, and then tell your mind to shut up.

Picture two separate entities:

1. You (the mind and personality that define you)

2. Your body (the machine that carries you around all the time and works its magic without you having to tell it what to do).

In yoga, we practice bringing the mind and body together. But my yoga class is virtually the only time I want my mind and body speaking for each other. My mind is the reason I got fat. My mind is the reason I fell off every diet I'd ever tried. It wasn't my body craving french fries and ice cream. It was my mind!

Few individuals truly honor their bodies enough to listen to them. They feel a mild pang of hunger and assume the body is asking for food. Or the office clock says it's lunch time and they assume the body wants to eat. If they took the time to ask their bodies, however, and really listen to the answer, they'd probably find out their bodies really aren't hungry at noon. Or the hunger pang is just part of the digestion process and doesn't mean the stomach must be fed. We think we know our bodies; yet, our organs constantly do utterly amazing things of which we have little personal understanding or appreciation. While we're rushing off to work, thinking about the tasks that lie ahead of us, the body is busy doing its own thing—digesting breakfast, cleansing the blood, and processing the air we breathe. We take it for granted that the body will do these things, just as we take it for granted that our car engine will start when we turn the key each morning.

We often identify with our bodies based solely on our feelings about them, rather than on fact or knowledge. Consider the anorexic who says, "I am fat." Her body may be emaciated, but her mind "feels" fat; therefore, she speaks--incorrectly--for her body. An undiagnosed cancer patient may say, "I'm fine and healthy," even while a tumor grows in her abdomen. Again, the person is speaking--out of turn--for the body.

Has this ever happened to you? You're talking with John and Jane. Jane asks *you* a question, and John *answers it for you*. It's rather irksome, isn't it? After all, you can speak up for yourself.

Your body can speak for itself too. You simply need to learn to ask questions of it, and then learn to listen. Notice again: I'm separating the "you" from your body.

Right now I'm sensing mild hunger, the kind you feel right before lunch. It starts in my stomach and seems to rise up the esophagus to the back of my mouth. My mind tells me I'm hungry. My mind is trying to tell me that my mouth, esophagus and stomach would feel better if I ate something. Yet I had a small breakfast a few hours ago, followed by a cup of Greek yogurt just 45 minutes ago. Already I've consumed plenty of nutrition in 230 calories. I'm not about to keel over from hunger. I don't even feel light-headed. Do I really need more food right now? I ask my body, directing my silent question to that big mass of bone, skin and organs that sits below my head. The answer my body gives me is surprising:

"I'm doing just fine, thank you. Unless you're planning to take an energetic two-mile walk right now, I don't need anything. All systems are functioning quite well. Check back in a few hours. Meanwhile, I could always stand a glass of water."

With an answer like that, I can let go of the idea that I MUST eat something to stay alive or even stay sane through the afternoon. My body, not my mind, has told me that food isn't necessary at the moment. Granted, my mind will keep poking at me, saying," Hey! Feed the body. Stuff the pie hole. You'll die if you don't!" But I can check with the body down below and confirm what it told me earlier: that everything's fine, all systems are "go," and that it needs nothing but would appreciate a glass of water. When I do check back later, I'll ask my body what it needs. It may tell me, "I need some protein," or "I could use a few quick carbs." It will even tell me how much Greek yogurt I should dish out.

Wouldn't it be nice to have a personal nutrition coach? Someone who can counsel you all day long and advise you on exactly what you need to eat? Someone with whom you can dialog about your eating habits and desires? Someone to prepare and serve all your meals to you? Well, you do have "someone" who can do it all. Again, it's your body. Start a new, respectful relationship with it. Not only will it tell you what *not* to eat, but it will tell you what it *needs* and when it's *had enough.* Next time you're tempted to cram a bag of chips down your esophagus, check in with your stomach and ask how it feels about all that crud getting piled in there. Learn to respect its wishes.

One of the best "diet" books I've ever read was "Diets Don't Work," by Bob Schwartz. It was a best-seller back in 1982. Schwartz followed it up with "Diets Still Don't Work," published in 1990. The follow-up reminded me of some of the great concepts he'd introduced in the first book, like "Rating Your Hunger." He encourages people to rate their hunger on a scale of 1 to 10. "**One** is when you're so hungry you feel faint. **Ten** is when you're so stuffed you can hardly move," he writes. Schwartz advises asking your body how hungry it is, and then rating it. **Unless it's under 5, don't eat.** Your body simply doesn't want or need it. Thin people, he says, eat only when they're hungry, and they stop eating when they're no longer hungry.

If you have trouble with portion control—and that's still my biggest downfall—eat more slowly. Take smaller bites and thoroughly chew each morsel. I know you've heard this so many times already that you want to throw up...but it really is true. Eating more slowly will give your stomach the chance to process the intake and to message you when it's full. To receive the message, of course, you must be listening. So tune in. As soon as your gut knows you're open to dialogue, it will tell you exactly what it needs and when. And the listening will get easier and easier.

As much as my mind loves fresh-baked bread and warm oatmeal cookies, my body tells me it can't tolerate them. I gave up gluten, oatmeal, bananas, peanuts, and a long list of other common foods because my gut told me it couldn't handle them. If I ignored my body's pleadings and ate my old favorite peanut butter and banana sandwich on whole wheat bread, I'd pay the price with gas, cramps and irregularity for the next 36 hours. My body doesn't lie to me! I'm finally learning to listen and trust that it knows what's best for me.

I ran this by my friend Laurie, and here's what she said:

"Okay, but I don't have those food sensitivity problems. I just like to eat. It feels good while I'm doing it, and not that bad afterward, except that I'm full....and as fat as ever."

Here's what I told her:

"Then I think you don't really know what 'feeling good' means, and that's a shame. If you feel 'normal' after eating the wrong foods or a little too much of anything, then it's because *feeling bad has become the norm for you.* And if you actually liked that feeling, you wouldn't be reading this book right now." It's like hitting your head with a hammer. If you do it day in and day out, the pain becomes "normal." If, however, you once realize how good you can feel when you stop, you'll never hit your head with another hammer.

Have conversations with your body, as if it's a separate entity from your mind.

Take its advice if it tells you that it would just as soon go to bed hungry tonight. Believe it if it tells you it would rather not have a bag of salty chips, or that it really doesn't want that second beer. Getting to know your own body, through conversation and listening, is the way to discover the thin person inside you.

Your body doesn't want to be heavy, after all. By good design, most of us aren't born fat. The average birth weight for a healthy baby is 6 to 9 pounds. If you're a typical overweight adult, you gained weight because of your lifestyle. Now your body is begging you to lighten it up, to remove stress from knee and hip joints, to allow it to move the way it was designed to move.

Once you begin sculpting away the fat and shaping your body into what you truly want, you will want to move even more. Success Breeds Success. The lighter and more toned you feel, the more you'll want to move. So keep moving. Any movement is exercise, and exercise burns calories. It's also a magic potion for feeling younger. As if that weren't good enough, the more muscle you gain back, the faster your resting metabolism will be. That means you can burn more calories than normal, even while you're sitting at your desk.

When we're carrying around a lot of extra fat, it's hard to get in touch with the body because it's covered in adipose tissue, like the white marshmallowy skin that encases a chocolate cake "snowball." We can't even see the body for the fat! We can't see the bones, the organs, the tendons, ligaments and muscle. We can't even see the true "naked" shape of our body as it was originally designed to look. It's no wonder we don't feel in touch with it. In fact, you may feel downright alienated from it. After all, how many times have you disgustedly grabbed a roll of fat at your waist or on your thighs and felt nothing but malice for that alien substance that had taken hold of your body? At that point, your body was the enemy. No wonder you felt like punishing it by feeding it even more! Overeating, or eating things you know are bad for it, are not loving acts of kindness toward the body that has kept you going all these years.

79

But as you start to lose that outer marshmallowy layer of fat, you'll see a structural frame emerging. You'll see hip bones, rib cage, and quadricep leg muscles revealing themselves. You will be amazed at the unveiling of your own structure, and you'll have a much greater appreciation of the hard-working body you've taken for granted, or possibly even abused, for so long. The body lying below the fat is your friend, not an adversary. Let it emerge!

Strike up a new camaraderie with this wonderful machine that is you, and let it tell you what it wants and needs to stay healthy. Once your body starts communicating its wishes to you, keep your mouth shut and listen. We tend to be butt-inskis when our bodies are speaking to us. If it starts to say, "I need carbs," let it finish the thought without you interrupting. We're used to doing that, you know. The body says, "I need food," and we think that grants us license to unbridled cravings. Just because the thought of pizza enters your head and sticks there like an obsession doesn't mean your body needs pizza. So don't push it! Dig a little deeper and ask your body what it really desires. Your mind wants pizza, but your body may actually want water, sleep, or even a cold diet soda instead. If your body does indeed insist on pizza, it may be in need of salt, a little extra fat, and some carbs. Go ahead and have the darn pizza; just eat it slowly and savor it. Drink lots of water after the first piece, and wait a few minutes before having a second piece. You'll have less room and less desire for it. Personally, I'd probably eat the second piece too, but I'd stop there because if I ate any more I'd be uncomfortable. Two pieces of pizza aren't going to destroy you. In fact, it may keep you satisfied for many hours! Contrast this approach to the old one--you know, where you order the pizza on late-night impulse and devour most of it immediately by yourself before you retire to bed?

BLWL Concept 3: "Handling depression"

If you're depressed and feeling miserable or angry, eating will only make it worse. Vent your frustrations another way. Later, you might still feel depressed, miserable and angry, but you will also be THINNER, which will make you feel smug, and eventually much better. Feeling angry/thinner is much better than feeling angry/fatter.

Many of us eat when we're depressed, bored, lonely, or frustrated. We grab food as if it's a drug to treat these emotional maladies—and it is, of course, for the moment. The sensations of chewing and tasting will temporarily take our mind off our problems for the few seconds we're eating it. But then, within minutes, we'll feel even worse than we did before we ate because now, on top of the depression, boredom, loneliness or frustration, we add self-loathing, guilt and helplessness. And if that weren't bad enough, we also just made ourselves heavier, which accelerates the whole downward spiral. We probably even gave ourselves a stomach ache. Now we're depressed, bored, lonely, frustrated and helpless, but we're also fatter and our tummies hurt. Suddenly, this "drug" of M&Ms, chips, macaroni and cheese, peanuts, or whatever you're ingesting for "comfort" doesn't sound so wonderful, does it? This type of food, eaten in these circumstances, is a drug that makes your original symptoms worse, not better.

Sometimes life just sucks. And it's not really because we're fat. It sucks because people can be mean, or because we make bad choices, or because it rains on the day we planned a picnic. Whatever the reason, we all have bad days, and some of us have more bad days than good.

But you know what? Even if we eat the wrong stuff in our quest to make things better, it's still going to be a bad day for the same reasons it started out that way. And it will be a whole lot worse if we make ourselves fatter in the process. If today was bad, tomorrow may be even worse (how's that for optimism?). But it won't be nearly as bad if you're skinnier tomorrow than you were today!

So go ahead and be mad at the world once in a while. Throw a fit, punch a pillow, cuss and mutter if you want. Just don't EAT to try to make it better, because the eating won't work. It will only make it worse. Being a grouchy size 6 is a lot better than being a grouchy size 16.

BLWL Concept 4: "Hunger is good"
Go to bed hungry. You'll fall asleep, you'll wake up without hunger, and you'll be thinner! Rule of thumb: the growlier your stomach is at bedtime, the better you will feel in the morning.

Most weight-reducing programs advise you to stop eating at least four hours before you go to bed. That means closing up the kitchen at 7 p.m., assuming you turn in at 11:00. That's hard if you're accustomed to having a cookie two hours after dinner, or a nightcap in front of the fire, or a little snack while finishing up your email. It may also be difficult for you to "embrace hunger." It's not natural for us to seek hunger and relish it. Our survival instincts tell us that hunger is a bad thing. Yet very few of us have ever known true hunger (malnourishment) or stayed even mildly hungry very long. It goes against our nature. After all, if we don't eat, we may just waste away.

Wait a minute! "Waste away"....isn't that what we'd like to do, figuratively speaking? Aha...so "hunger" means we are losing weight! Hey, suddenly hunger pangs become *pleasant* sensations!

Granted, this may be a difficult mindset adjustment for you to make if you're accustomed to grabbing "emergency rations" the minute you feel signs of hunger. Again, converse with your body and it will tell you that the sensations of hunger aren't such a bad thing, especially before bed. Your body will rest much better on an empty stomach than on a full one. In other words, you'll get a better night's sleep and wake up refreshed. Not only that, but you will NOT feel hungry when you jump out of bed in the morning! The hunger will return after you're up and moving, but that will give you sufficient time to feel thinner (a great way to start the day!), weigh yourself, and maybe even try on a clothing item that was snug the day before. By starting out the day as a thinner person, you'll be better able to maintain the momentum throughout the rest of the day. You'll have more optimism and confidence about your ability to control your food intake, and will actually look forward to bedtime hunger and waking up lighter.

Initially, pre-bedtime hunger may actually provide you with more energy, making it harder for you to "wind down" for sleep. Here's a no-calorie solution: have a glass of water, take a warm bath or shower, have another glass of water, and then GO TO BED! You'll eventually go to sleep (it usually happens sooner than you think it will). You'll probably wake up at least once to get rid of all that water you drank before bed, but you will not be hungry. Keep a water glass by the sink and have another sip or two before you return to bed. Again, when you wake up in the morning, you won't have any immediate sense of hunger.

Think about the last time you overate--or just ate anything high in calories--right before you went to bed. Your first waking thoughts were something like, "Oh my god, I ate six brownies before bed last night. I am such a loser. I'm fatter this morning than I was yesterday." You're starting out your day with negativity, which can spiral you (and everyone around you) into a pit as the day wears on. Wouldn't it be better to wake up "empty," thinner, energized, and with a positive self image? That's a wave you can ride for the next 24 hours!

A few people have told me that they simply can't sleep if they're hungry. I disagree. They may be restless the first night, but the physical sensation of "hunger" passes as the digestive system adjusts to less work. Ask anyone who's fasted; they'll tell you most physical feelings of hunger pass within a day or so.

I'm no sleep expert, and I rarely get insomnia. But when I do, I usually force myself to stay in bed and simply meditate. Even if I'm not particularly sleepy, I know I'm resting my mind and body. As relaxation comes, so will sleep.

On those very rare occasions when I wake up at 3 a.m. and can't get back to sleep, it's generally because of other pain issues—a sore back, a stiff hip, aching shoulders resulting from too much activity the day before. If discomforts compels you to get up at night and stay up for a while, try reading or internet shopping for clothing in the smaller sizes you'll soon be wearing. Keep away from food sources. After all, why would you want to shove food down your throat in the middle of the night? Your body neither wants nor needs it when it's in resting mode.

BLWL Concept 5: "Calorie tally"
Keep a running tally of your calories. You'll find no need to "throw in the towel" for the day just because you fell off the wagon and ate three cookies. You may still be well within your range of 1000-1200 calories a day.

No matter what weight-loss drugs or other treatments you may have resorted to, it all still gets down to simple physics: If you want to lose weight, you have to eat fewer calories than you burn. Consume more than you can burn, and you "save" the extras in your body's fat bank, which is usually on your butt or around your belly.

My mom actually had it right when she painstakingly made her daily food lists and tucked them inside her "Joy of Cooking" copy 50 years ago.

Women in my age group--51 and over--need between 1600 and 2200 calories a day to maintain their weight. The exact number depends, of course, on their activity levels. Sedentary women may need fewer than 1600, and women training for triathlons will need more than 2200. In order to lose fat, we must consume fewer calories than our maintenance level requires. An accepted rule of thumb is to reduce your calorie intake by at least 500, but not more than 1000, below your maintenance level. The American College of Sports Medicine recommends that calorie levels never drop below 1200 calories per day for women or 1800 calories per day for men.

Well, okay, but I discovered that I need considerably less if I'm going to lose weight. It took me weeks of monitoring my weight and calorie intake to discover the right number of calories for me. If I want to lose weight, I can't eat any more than 1000 to 1100 calories a day. That's what got my weight off. Now I maintain my weight by eating between 1000 and 2500. Discovering my own personal "magic number" makes it easy for me to fall back into a weight loss pattern in case I let a few pounds creep back onto my thighs.

Former supermodel Christie Brinkley consumes about 1100 calories in an average day. She's now in her late 50s and weighs about 135 pounds. I'm sure even the perfect Miss Brinkley has some moments of food insanity, but she knows that 1100 calories is her healthy limit if she's going to maintain her supermodel body. Is it difficult? Probably not for her. She's a vegetarian and has had many years of practice eating "lite" and "healthy."

Here's the point: no matter what the charts may tell you, it's up to you to find your own caloric balance between losing/maintaining/gaining weight. Some sources claim a woman should never eat less than 1200 calories a day if she's to stay sufficiently nourished. But Christie Brinkley, at 5'9", looks pretty darned healthy. So don't necessarily use the "expert's" advice as an excuse to lose at a slower pace than you find satisfying and healthy. We're all individuals with different metabolisms.

If you haven't already become calorie-savvy, do so. It's ridiculously easy to find the calorie content of any food these days. Never mind that there are hundreds of calorie-counting books in publication. Just look up a food on the internet and you'll find the often startling numbers within seconds. Take "Costco Four-Cheese Ravioli," for instance. Google it and you'll find the nutritional information at several different sources. That way, if you lose the label for a product, you can look it up instantly on the internet and find out, for instance, that the 12 little leftover ravioli pillows you ate for lunch today mounted up to nearly 500 calories…and a lot of sodium, to boot.

Let's say you didn't intend to eat that leftover ravioli at all because you just knew it was too high in calories for you. But you cave in because it's there in front of you in the fridge, and you don't want it to go bad and, besides, you need the energy because you didn't have much for breakfast.

So you start eating this ravioli, left over from last night's dinner, and you intend to only have three or four. But before you know it, you've sucked down all 12. Now you really feel miserable because you're sure you've totally blown your eating regimen for the whole day. And since you've already blown it, you might as well keep going and eat the leftover garlic bread too…and a chunk of cheese from the Parmesan wedge….and why not have several cookies too, since today is a lost cause!

Hold it!! Assuming you had a modest breakfast--let's say some fruit and a huge glob of no-fat Greek yogurt--and then you ate 12 ravioli, you've still only ingested about 750 calories. Granted, that doesn't leave you much wiggle room for dinner. But 750 calories is still way under your daily limit, and it's now mid-afternoon. You still have a chance to salvage the day, or at least not sabotage the rest of it with unrestrained eating. If you eat another 400 calories between now and bedtime, you're still doing just fine. Much better than if you'd thrown in the towel after the ravioli and consumed another 900 calories in frustration!

You want to eat a bag of chips? Fine, do it. Just look at the calorie count on the back of the bag and realize you'll be stuffing 600-900 calories down your gullet. If you do that, you'd better not plan on eating much else that day. Prepare to feel lousy too, because that's just not a good plan for getting your nutritional needs met. But the point is this: count the calories as you are consuming them, and you will still be in control. If you stop counting because you think you were a bad, despicable loser for eating those chips, you'll end up ingesting hundreds or even thousands more calories by day's end. After all, you can always re-start your wise eating tomorrow, right? Yes, that's right, and you'll also be spending the next several days burning off the extra fat you crammed into your body after you ate the chips.

You can't "undo" the chips by eating more balanced foods on top of them. But if you try to apologize to your body by eating a well rounded meal on top of the chips, you're only going to feel worse and you will have packed in even more unnecessary calories. If you ate the chips, it's best to cut your losses and try to maintain the rest of your calorie count at the daily level that works best for you.

Shock away your desire
Personally I'm glad to see all the "Nutrition Facts" on food packaging these days. It's helped me walk away from many an otherwise appealing item on the grocer's shelf. Even when I've been insanely, dangerously hungry and have felt reckless enough to buy and eat without restraint, I suddenly lose my desire when I read the back of a snack bag and find out a whole bag of this popcorn-like product contains 2400 calories. I know darn well if I bought the bag, I'd eat the whole thing and not the "single serving" that's microscopic in size. Do I really want to be tempted with an open bag of snacks that's got 2400 calories concentrated into just a few ounces? No, thank you! Back on the shelf it goes.

You always hear about how you'll have to jog for half an hour to burn off one small Hershey Bar. Or how you'll have to climb stairs for 15 minutes to burn off a small cookie. But I never eat just one small cookie. And if there's a bag of my favorite candy--Skittles--nearby, I'm not going to stop at 10 pieces (40 calories). I'll want to eat at least a cupful. That's 830 calories of sugar and chemicals I could mindlessly devour as I'm sitting at the computer or driving on a road trip. If it's an all-day drive, I could probably eat twice that many. Ouch...that's 1660 calories, just from candy. Theoretically, if I'm counting calories, that means I couldn't eat anything at all for the next day and a half. I think I'll opt for something else to keep me alert...like maybe a huge coffee with just a smidgeon of nonfat creamer...or some sugar-free gum...or an energy shot...or just plain old water. I definitely have choices, and when a "Nutrition Facts" label slaps me in the face with a high calorie count, it's a lot easier to make the right choices.

Read the label BEFORE you buy the product. It will probably dissuade you from buying it at all. This type of prevention is proactive and it keeps you in control, which is good for your psyche. Contrast this to the "Jog 30 minutes to burn off a small candy bar," and you immediately see the difference. The latter approach is reactive, which means you're on the defense; you're trying to fix something that went wrong. Being proactive and being in control is much more fun and much kinder to your self image.

Familiarize yourself with the caloric content of some of your most favorite go-to foods. I love plain nonfat Greek yogurt, and I know I can eat a whole huge tub of it a day and only ingest 560 calories. I love red grapes and eat as many as I want when they're in season. A cup of grapes has just 110 calories, and that's really a lot of grapes. A frozen boneless skinless chicken breast also has about 110 calories. Hard-boiled eggs:

70 calories each. An Alaskan Summer Ale: 158. A small package of M&Ms: 240 calories. That's quite a few...but if I want chocolate, I'll eat it and just put it in my running tally for the day. Allowing myself the occasional treat isn't at all out of the question. And just because I eat chocolate doesn't mean I'm going to give up on the rest of the day and punish myself by eating whatever is in front of me.

A typical day for me might be like this:

- A third of a tub of Greek yogurt: 200 calories

- Water and coffee

- Hard-boiled egg: 70 calories

- More water

- Strawberries from the garden: 40 calories

- More Greek yogurt: 200 calories

- Glass of white wine: 125 calories

- More water

- Chicken breast: 110 calories

- Second glass of wine: 125 calories

- Hommus wrapped in lettuce leaves

- More water

- A big bunch of grapes: 200 calories

Total calories: 1070

And a variation:

- Water and coffee

- Brown rice and scrambled egg mixed together

- More water

- Grapes

- Yogurt

- Small package of M&Ms

- Water

- Wine

- Huge green salad with leftover chicken mixed in

- More water

Just glancing at this, I know it will be well under my 1200-calorie limit, and will satisfy my body. If I'm "bad" and have a second glass of wine and a few more grapes, I'll still be okay.

Personally, I am most comfortable with eating between 400 and 500 calories during the day (before 5 p.m.) and using my balance for an evening meal and an alcoholic beverage.

Nutritionally...no lectures, please. I take a multi-vitamin supplement, fish oil, calcium citrate, and Vitamin E (the real one here, not Excedrin). I get tons of protein and calcium from my diet, plenty of fiber, very little fat, and very few processed foods containing lots of sodium and chemicals. No breads, no potatoes, no bananas, no whole grains, no dairy (except Greek yogurt and small amounts of hard cheeses) very limited amounts of tomatoes and citrus fruits. This may sound nuts to you, but it's an eating lifestyle that works for me. *You have to develop your own, by finding the foods that satisfy you while nourishing you, and by listening to your body for advice on when and how much to eat.*

About alcohol.....
Of course you can include it if you can handle it. Just remember the four ways alcohol can sabotage your weight-loss efforts:

1. It removes your inhibitions and "happies" you up so you will probably eat more without caring at the time.

2. It is ridiculously high in calories. Figure roughly 100 calories per ounce of hard liquor (gin, whiskey, vodka). An ounce isn't very much booze, so you'll probably want more. It's easy to pour 600 calories or more of zero-nutrition alcohol and mixed drinks (yes, don't forget to count the calories in the mixes) down your throat during an evening.

3. It is often served with salty snacks. The salt will cause water retention, and you won't like that when you get on the scale the next morning.

4. You're more likely to drink alcohol at night, which means you're consuming all those liquid calories, plus the predictable munchies, right before bed when your metabolism is about to slow down. That means you may wake up heavier than you were before the alcohol consumption.

Alcohol is, without a doubt, my biggest stumbling block. I like my wine, beer, margarita, or brandy most evenings. But when I drink, my food-related willpower and common sense fly out the window. So the most effective strategy I've developed is to enjoy my cocktail earlier in the evening, say an hour before dinner, and drink plenty of water alongside the spirits. That fills me up while leaving room for a light dinner, after which the kitchen and bar are closed up tight for the evening. I don't drink every evening, and I am acutely aware that my weigh-in the next morning is always better when I don't have alcohol the night before.

BLWL Concept 6: "Weighing in"
Weigh EVERY day to keep yourself on track and to learn about (and accept) your body's natural fluctuations.

Do you fear and loathe the scale? I bet you and I have both played the same "scale games," like these:

- Be stark naked when you weigh, which includes removing your post earrings.

- Go to the bathroom and wring out your bladder as thoroughly as possible prior to weighing.

- Don't weigh unless you've pooped first.

- Don't weigh if you overate last night.

- Don't weigh if you think you're retaining water for whatever reason.

- Work out for an hour beforehand.

- Don't weigh if you're already depressed.

- Step gingerly onto the scale so there's no "bounce effect."

- Carefully shift your feet around on the scale until it reads as low as possible.

- Step off and try the whole process again.

- Go the bathroom once more before you try weighing for the third time.

- Make sure there's no one around to see you (naked or not).

- Fast all day and then weigh yourself at 5:00 when your stomach is empty and you're dehydrated.

- Avoid the scale altogether and embrace the concept that "It's how your clothes fit, not what the scale measures, that's important."

Sounds kind of silly, doesn't it? How can we get so tightly wound about stepping on a mechanical thing that registers our body weight? Maybe it's because that brainless-therefore-objective thing slaps us in the face with reality. It rockets us out of our pleasant residence in the State of Denial and plops us down hard like a sack of moon rocks. As long as we don't know how much we weigh, we can imagine we're 20 pounds lighter than we actually are.

The difference here, between Denial and Reality, is that we can fool our minds but we can't fool our bodies. Once again, the two seem to reside in different time zones. You know you're overweight, but your mind reassures you that you're not THAT overweight. The mind is so persuasive in its argument that it gives you permission to eat more, to enjoy one more binge, to "live life to the fullest" (by indulging), and to put off the diet until tomorrow. That's how you stay fat for the rest of your life. And while your mind convinces you that you're not "that" overweight," your joints still know the truth as they ache and strain under the unnecessary fat.

But what if I told you that the mere act of stepping on the scale, especially if you haven't done it for a while, **is the first positive step toward guaranteed *Bucket List Weight Loss*?** Your experience with the scale will actually jump-start the process, almost as dramatically as taking one of those old-fashioned diet pills (i.e. "speed.") Once you establish your starting point--what the scale says you weigh today--and then consistently monitor your weight, you're going to experience an automatic behavior change so subtle that you won't even know it's happening at first. Your appetite will decrease. You'll start looking at food in a different way. You won't be obsessing about eating. Your energy will increase. Your attitude will become more optimistic. You will feel emotionally and physically stronger. Even if you're not consciously trying to change your eating and activity habits, your heightened awareness of body weight will start causing a weight loss. This is because you have started listening to your body and acknowledging its reality, rather than listening to your mind and living in a fantasy world that ends at your neck.

Getting over Scale Phobia

Stepping onto a scale, when you're overweight and haven't been on a scale for a long time because you've avoided it, is about as scary as bungee jumping. At least it's been that way for me. Even as a Size 6, it's still a cliff-hanging moment. It gets easier and much less dramatic as you do it more frequently, and the initial shock of the first weighing goes away as soon as you settle into reality and accept the fact that you are what you are today. If you still dread stepping on the scale that first time after a long absence from it, try this to help prepare you for the results:

First, wait until you're feeling terrific about yourself. Maybe you just had a super-successful day at work and you feel invincible. Maybe you bought a terrific new outfit that makes you look hot. Maybe you just got a new hairdo, or changed your makeup, and you love what you see in the mirror. In fact, you're looking pretty darn good all over, and you feel like you have the world by the tail. Even the most depressed people have occasional bouts of optimism, and that's when you want to seize the moment to boldly weigh yourself.

Now, with that very positive self image in your head, step onto a scale you trust. Don't try to guess what the results will be. Just look down and objectively accept what the scale tells you, as if you're a nurse weighing someone in a clinic.

Are you surprised with the results? Study the numbers for a moment, and then step off the scale. Now immediately recall how good you felt about yourself 30 seconds earlier. Remind yourself that you're still that same successful, confident, attractive person. The fact that you now know how much that person weighs should have little or no bearing on how you feel about yourself. NOTHING ABOUT YOU HAS CHANGED in the last 30 seconds!

You now have a starting point; the mystery you've dreaded solving is over. Now you can get on with your weight loss, knowing you'll just look and feel THAT MUCH BETTER as the excess weight begins to melt away. And, like any new endeavor, the more you weigh yourself, the easier and less "personal" it will seem. It might even become something you look forward to; as you see the numbers start to drop.

Have you ever felt embarrassed when the nurse weighs you prior to a medical appointment? You're probably thinking, "Oh no, she must be shocked to see someone who weighs so much. My secret is out! She's forming her opinion of me right now, and she'll remember this moment forever!"

Whoa! That nurse probably weighed 30 people today, some undoubtedly larger than you. She's rushed, she's stressed, and she probably isn't even paying any lasting attention to your name or your face. She's recording your weight on a chart, with automatic efficiency. She doesn't CARE how much you weigh. All she wants to do is write down a number on paper and get you into an exam room so she can go retrieve the next person from the waiting room.

You are not the heaviest person in the world. There's a good chance the person who just weighed you weighs more than you, and that everyone in the waiting room weighs more than you. That's a sad commentary on society these days, but it's possible. Most people probably weigh more than you think they do. Most people have the same loathing for their fat stomachs, butts and thighs. Most people don't care about the exact number you just registered on the scale, because they're too concerned about their own numbers.

Remember those people if your scale phobia returns. Realize that they might like to be you, instead. You, after all, are reading this book so you're about to get control of your weight issue for good. They don't have that yet. They're still very overweight, with no compass to guide them to thinness. The number you see when you step onto the scale is not a reflection of who you are as a person. It merely tells you how much stress you're putting on your knees, hips, feet, and back. Armed with that information, you now know what you must change to decrease your joint pain, aid your mobility and flexibility, and make yourself look 10 years younger.

From now on, you're going to weigh every day.

But what if everyone says you should only weigh once a week? Well, lots of popular weight-loss programs suggest weighing only once a week. Their reasoning? If you weigh more often, you'll get discouraged by the normal fluctuations I just mentioned. If you weigh more often, you may become unhealthfully obsessed with your weight. (Obsessions generally aren't good things.)

However, I advocate weighing every day (same time of day, same clothing). *It keeps you accountable for your daily actions.* I've known many Weight Watchers and TOPS (Take Off Pounds Sensibly) devotees who will fall "off the wagon" for a few days during the week, and then fast at the last minute before their weekly weigh-ins at meetings. This behavior reinforces the very eating habits that caused the weight gain to begin with. Starve the day before weigh-in, then binge the day after. These people are basically daring their scales, and their programs, that they can eat without conscience immediately after weighing, and then fix their transgressions by fasting before their next weigh-in. Granted, not everyone involved in such weekly weigh-in programs plays the game to an extreme like this. But enough do that it bears mentioning. These people are practicing an obsessive/compulsive behavior that does nothing to foster a long-term, healthy, and permanent weight loss.

To establish good habits that you can practice EVERY day, you must be held accountable EVERY day. Weighing EVERY day can do that. When you vow to step on the scale every morning, you are less likely to splurge on pizza and ice cream the night before.

Becoming accountable for your own actions is the first step toward controlling them. Quite simply, a daily weigh-in will help keep you honest.

Prepare for mystery fluctuations
Sometimes I'll gleefully jump onto the scale in the morning, fully expecting to see a significant drop because I was so "good" the day before. Instead, the scale tells me I've gained two pounds since yesterday! What the bleep!! I'll shake my head, cuss again, and try stepping on for a second opinion. Well, darn, it says the same thing as last time; I'm up two pounds. At that point I may just shake my head, roll my eyes, and accept the mysterious reality; my body really does seem to manufacture weight from air!

But of course it doesn't. So I'll rack my brain and mentally retrace yesterday's footsteps, trying to figure out what I ate that caused a two-pound weight gain. Sometimes I can't come up with any explanation, not even water retention, although that usually is what it is. I simply have to accept that the body is doing weird things, holding onto weird little pockets of water somewhere--water I didn't even know I had in me--and that it will flush it all out when the body is good and ready. My job is to wait, to stay the course, and to remain patient.

That's why I advocate weighing daily, not just once a week as many diet programs dictate.

Wouldn't it be discouraging to go to your weekly TOPS meeting and get the surprising news that you'd gained two pounds since last week's weigh-in? At that point it doesn't matter that you'll probably lose the two pounds of water by tomorrow morning. The meeting is tonight.

If you only weigh once a week, you're not as aware of those natural fluctuations, and you're not as mentally or emotionally prepared to handle them. The shock of learning you'd "gained" two pounds, when you were anticipating a loss, may be enough to send you into a tailspin of defeatist thinking that could also lead to inappropriate eating. ("What the hell, I might as well just give up and eat a bunch of junk food...")

In this scenario, the scale becomes your nemesis.

On the other hand, weighing daily on your own, under consistent conditions, will allow you to *emotionally* divorce yourself from the Almighty Scale. You'll learn to use it as an insightful tool to spy on your body and get to know it better. While you do, keep reminding yourself of this fact: the body will lose fat if you burn more calories than you consume. Period. It may be a slow process, but it will work. Guaranteed. It will come off if you're doing everything else right. Best of all, it will stay off.

Concentrate on today

In the meantime, as you're waiting (impatiently) for the scale to drop, go ahead and enjoy life! You are, after all, probably thinner than you were yesterday or last week. This is a wonderful thing! Gradually start tuning in to your new body. Notice how your energy has increased, your joints don't ache all the time, and you're able to stand just a little straighter and prouder. Even breathing is probably becoming easier. Rather than setting your sights on a weight-loss goal date (like your daughter's wedding, or a class reunion), concentrate on enjoying life as a thinner person *today*. The "one day at a time" adage applies here. But instead of looking at weight-loss as a daily *struggle*, consider it a daily *challenge!*

Don't shoot the scale...or yourself

Let's say you're having some success with daily weighings. Then you splurge on a hefty dinner and two margaritas. The next morning the scale says you've gained four pounds. What should you do? Laugh! You can swear at the scale too, if you want, but then laugh again! The scale isn't telling you that you're fat! It's just letting you know that your body is going through normal fluctuations, probably related to water retention. You didn't put on four pounds of fat last night.

Granted, it's discouraging to see those spikes on the weight chart when we desperately want to see a consistent loss. But you MUST keep the faith! *Accept the fact that you're not going to lose 20 pounds by next week.* Your weight will fluctuate, seemingly without explanation, maybe in a five-pound range as you are slowly and steadily burning fat. Your body has its own rhythms and frequently "does its own thing," regardless of what our emotions want it to do.

BUCKET LIST WEIGHT LOSS

Weighing DAILY will help you come to terms with this natural process, and become more accepting and understanding of the body in which you reside.

Choose your scale with care!
I've always had a hard time trusting a mechanical scale with a spring in it. You step on with one foot, then immediately step off and watch the needle boomerang back two pounds light. Then you adjust the little tension wheel on it, and the next time it weighs two pounds heavy. When you're actually ready to go for the full weight, you step on it very gingerly, one foot at a time, easing down onto it ever so slowly and taking great care to make sure the needle doesn't bounce way up and then rebound to an unreliable final figure.

Today's digital scales for home use may not be any more accurate, but at least they don't bounce. They settle on an irrefutable number and stay there. That's why I prefer to weigh on the "balance board" that comes with the Wii Fit program. There's a digital scale built into it. You set the balance board on the floor in front of your TV. The animated characters on the screen will tell you when to step on, and they talk you through the process of standing still and centered for a few seconds while the balance board registers your weight. The first reading it gives you is your BMI (Body Mass Index), which indicates the percentage of fat you're carrying. The BMI calculation is based on your height, build, gender and age--information which you enter into the Wii Fit program the very first time you start it.

The Wii will first display your BMI, and then offer you the chance to click on a separate button to see your actual weight. You don't have to look at it if you don't want to, but it will still record your weight and save it in a graph form so you can admire your progress later.   Being able to actually see the results on a graph is very reinforcing, since the cycles of ups and downs become so apparent. You'll see the spike and remember the big dinner with two margaritas. You'll see a big dip and recall how elated you were at the results that morning. Most of all, you'll see the steady loss of weight, objectively illustrated right there in front of you. That alone can be enough to motivate you to continue your new and better lifestyle...a lifestyle that includes *daily accountability through daily weighing*

BLWL Concept 7: "Move it"
Move! Keep your body in the perpetual motion it seeks.

The human body was designed for movement, not for being still. The muscles, bones, joints, ligaments and tendons want desperately to move, to stretch, to lubricate and massage themselves, and to stay in good operating order. They can't if you remain sedentary, whether you're thin or not.

When you sit still, you rust like the Tin Man. Your metabolism slows down, meaning you're not burning fat calories. Your mind gets fuzzy, your joints get stiff, and you start feeling really old, really fast.

Start moving as much as you can throughout the day. Walk, pace, stand at your computer instead of sitting. Take stairs; park the car a bit farther out in the lot than you normally do. Do knee bends or calf raises while you're pumping gas, or when you're riding alone in an elevator. Do isometric exercises at your desk. Stretch frequently. Keep grip strengtheners in your desk drawer. Dance in the kitchen while waiting for water to boil on the stove. Relish the opportunity to wash and vacuum floors, because these activities burn calories. Take the dog for two long walks a day. Spend time each day in a home gym or a health club.

I'm not suggesting you get out there and do an hour of cardio exercise every day, even though I try to do that myself. Sure, a heavy workout will burn calories and get rid of fat. But the movement I'm talking about is gentle and consistent throughout the day. Just don't sit still for long! Even if you do sit, try some isometric butt-tightening exercises, or do some bicep curls with a water bottle. Embrace any opportunity to move!

Movement will help you enjoy and appreciate the new body you've recently met. Like a new car, you'll want to drive it and marvel in its ability to get you places and do things for you. Movement will help you feel younger. As you slowly drop the pounds, movement won't hurt like it used to. One day you'll be going through your daily activities and will suddenly notice that nothing hurts anymore. Weight loss and movement are the best tonics for feeling good, and they cost virtually nothing.

So you don't like to sweat? Your mind tells you to stop moving as soon as you start breathing hard? You cease the movement when you get a burning sensation in your muscles? Unless you have a medical condition that truly precludes you from such movement, get used to it. This is what exercise is supposed to feel like. You will get sweaty as your body heats up with the physical stress. *This is natural, normal, and desirable.* When you start breathing hard, monitor your heart rate and keep it within the acceptable range for your age and body mass. The accepted rule of thumb for years has been **between 60 and 80% of 220 minus your age.** When you can no longer carry on a conversation while exercising, slow down and catch your breath until you can pass the "talk test." Then stick with that pace. If you feel a mild burning or aching sensation in your muscles, it's because you haven't used them for a while and they need work.

Moving your muscles burns calories. As an added benefit, moving your muscles can help them grow in mass. Muscles burn more calories than fat, even when they're at rest. So...the more muscle you have on your body, the faster you'll be burning calories, even when you're sitting around relaxing.

If you're physically limited
Unless you're 100% paralyzed or dead, there's always some type of exercise you can do to move your muscles. Isometrics can be done virtually anywhere by anyone, because they isolate and build strength in small, specific muscle groups. You don't need any special equipment and you don't even need to move. Pushing against a wall is a good example of an isometric exercise. Holding a dumbbell with your arm half-curled is another. Or try sitting in a chair, tensing your abdominal muscles, and raising your feet slightly off the floor. Hold any isometric pose for at least 10 seconds and you'll get a training benefit from it. Your muscles will strengthen and grow, and this will increase your metabolism....which means you'll burn calories faster, even when you're just resting.

When I was recovering from my four hip replacement surgeries, I was pretty limited in what I could do for exercise. But I didn't have to completely stop moving! I only had to protect the surgical area and not put stress on the new hip implant for a few weeks. So I gently worked other body parts while I mostly sat in a recliner in the living room. I was careful to isolate the muscles I was using so I could let the hip areas totally rest and recover. Even with those limitations, I did bicep curls, tricep isometrics (raising myself out of the chair using only my arm muscles), ankle rotations, and yoga-like stretches. My recovering body felt much better in careful movement than it did just sitting still and getting stiff.

If you're not sure what types of exercises are appropriate for your physical limitations, of course ask your doctor. Request physical therapy if it hasn't already been suggested. Make sure you communicate to your therapist that you want to work on all parts of your body, not just the parts that may need rehab due to your condition. Throughout my bouts of hip replacements, I've found that many doctors aren't particularly interested in the rehab/reconditioning phase of healing. If I've wanted more than the standard five days of outpatient PT following a surgery, I've had to ask for it. If your insurance won't allow PT follow-up that addresses all your body's needs, then Google your condition and seek information on your own regarding what types of exercises are appropriate for you. Following any restrictions your doctor may have given you, set up an exercise routine of your own. It will speed your recovery, help any chronic condition, give you a huge emotional boost, and dramatically speed up your weight reduction.

In other words, there is no excuse for not moving your body! And since it's no longer in vogue to roll your eyes and say, "I just hate exercise," you can't use that one either. So figure out how you're going to do it, and get started. Here are some suggestions.

Take your dog for a walk. As a dog trainer, I can attest that the best form of mental and physical exercise for your dog is leash-walking. Yes, leash-walking. Your dog doesn't have to run free to expend his energy. Plus, if you're on the other end of the leash, you'll be working hard too, which makes it a team event!

Get a Wii and play the interactive games on your TV. The Wii Fit and Wii Sports programs are tremendous, because you can play fitness games that are short in duration but heavy in results. With a few possible exceptions, the Wii activities are pretty gentle. Heck, that's why they're popular in nursing homes. You won't get a hot, heavy workout from any of them (with the possible exception of the hula hoop challenge, which whips my butt every time). Still, it's the duration of time you spend playing the games that adds up. Before you know it, the Wii timer will announce that you've been "working out" for 15 minutes. Play a few more self-challenging games of tennis, or swing few more bats to accumulate home runs, or spar a few more rounds with your boxing coach, and suddenly you've been moving for an hour--and having a great time! You're not sweaty, but you're warmed up and you've used some muscles.

My Wii Fit games and balance board will probably be obsolete in a few years, but they'll no doubt be replaced by an even more realistic and more effective type of interactive fitness program I can play on the TV screen. Already the market is flooded with workout DVDs for every level of fitness. Start with something gentle like Leslie Sansone's "Walk Away the Pounds" series, and increase your challenges to suit your improving fitness. Zumba and related forms of "total body" dancing are available on DVDs too, meaning you don't even have to leave your living room anymore to get a fantastic workout. (Wow, wouldn't Jack LaLanne be elated knowing what he started has come full circle!)

You can't dance because you have no toes? Then do the arm motions. Work your legs while sitting in a chair.

Tap your foot. Did you know you can burn 18 calories an hour just doing this? Some people call that nervous energy. I just call it a love of moving. I want to drive this machine that is my body just as far as I can and burn as much fuel as I can. I don't want an economy body that gets high mileage on very little fuel. I want a body that burns energy like crazy. And I get that through *movement.*

Take the damn stairs. Our laziness as a culture has conditioned us to always seek the parking space closest to the door, or stand around waiting for an elevator to take us up one story. Start parking a little farther out. Walk up the stairs. Movement is energizing, not energy draining! Need an analogy? Think of those little emergency flashlights you have to crank to produce a light. Your body's the same way. Move it, crank it, and it will produce something akin to the Fountain of Youth. Let it sit idle and it will deteriorate until it's a piece of junk.

Do the hard-core stuff. Find a cardio (heart-pumping) exercise you can stand to do at least three times a week for 30-40 minutes straight. It could be a Zumba DVD, a good treadmill, stair-climbing, fast walking, paddling a kayak, or bouncing on a mini-trampoline (aka rebounder). This will super-charge your weight loss. Believe me, you won't lose your Bucket List weight without some of this--or at least you may die of old age before you do. You may not like the sweatiness, the burning, and the labored breathing that are inherent with most types of exercise, but you will learn to embrace them and you may even experience the "runner's high," which is caused when your brain releases endorphins (natural pain killers) into your system. Most of the discomforts associated with exercise are transitory. As you get in better shape, you may even develop an addiction to workouts. While no addiction is healthy, it sure beats being addicted to ice cream and potato chips. Ask your *body* which it would prefer, and it will scream "Movement!" every time. Respect its opinion.

BLWL Concept 8: "Tummy knows best"

Don't eat something just because it's "good for you." If your body doesn't want it at the moment, don't eat it. Either eat NOTHING, or eat what your body really tells you it wants/ needs.

As you begin to feel better from the elimination of detrimental foods, your body will speak more loudly to you and overrule what your mind might demand you feed it. Let's say you haven't eaten for several hours, your daily calorie count is low, and you know you "should" eat something. You have broccoli, kale and spinach in the refrigerator, and it will go bad if you don't eat it soon. Your mind is telling you that you really should make a salad and eat these nutritious vegetables waiting for you in your crisper. But your body just can't get excited about it. So you ask your body what it would like to eat. After a few minutes of listening, you hear your body respond, "Canned corn."

"What the--!" your mind responds. "If you're going to be that way about it, I might as well just eat some tortilla chips." That's your mind interfering again. Tell your mind to shut up. If you just asked your body what it wants to eat, and it replied, "Canned corn," then open that little can of Niblets that's been sitting in your pantry for six months. Eat and enjoy. Don't let your conscience tell you that you're all wrong because you don't want to eat those greens that will be getting slimy soon.

Isn't it interesting how our mind--our conscience--can sabotage us with evil thoughts of junk food binges one minute, and then lay a guilt trip on us the next because we don't want to eat what it says we really should eat. All the more reason not to trust your mind to make food decisions. Listen to your body instead. It will tell you what it needs, when it needs it, and how much is enough.

So go for the Niblets today! Canned corn has 80 calories per half-cup. Granted, it's not as packed with nutrients as the greens, but it's not void of them either. And for some reason, your body tells you it wants to chew on those yellow kernels. Trust your cravings. They're coming from your body, not your head. For some strange reason your body needs corn today, so oblige it. *You will find yourself more satisfied with less food if you ask your body what it really wants and needs.*

Stop the regimented eating

I still cook two meals a day for my husband, and I used to feel guilty if I didn't sit down with him and eat a bit of whatever I cooked for him. That's over now. A typical dinner may be roast beef, brown rice, carrots, cornbread and salad, with rhubarb crisp for dessert. All of it's good and nutritious, but if I'm not hungry when I serve him, I won't eat most of that food and I may not eat anything. Usually I'd still sit down with him and enjoy a glass of wine or maybe a small amount of brown rice. I may have two pieces of carrot. I know they're practically no calories, but that makes no difference to me. If I don't really want them, I won't eat them.

For years I subscribed to the theory that breakfast must be eaten, whether you're hungry or not. No more. There will be days when I don't eat until early afternoon...not because I'm purposely trying to fast, but because I'm simply too busy to eat and food is a low priority on my list. It's because I'm listening to my body, rather than letting my mind pick up food cues from the world around me. Usually around mid-afternoon on such days, I'll start feeling a little light-headed, indicating my blood sugar is low. Then I'll eat something high in protein and easy to digest, like a hard-boiled egg or some Greek yogurt. Never again do I want to "crash" as I did that day at the YMCA after my sauna, fast, and blood donation!   Water can be a renovating elixir as well. Within minutes I'll have the energy to carry on, and the satisfaction of knowing I haven't overstepped my calorie boundaries for the day.

Countless diet programs still encourage us to carry baggies of raw carrots and celery, or little boxes of raisins, to help us through days when we're denying ourselves what we really want to eat. I have yet to find a raw carrot or even an apple as truly satisfying as a few crackers with peanut butter, or even a small bag of M&Ms. Granted, you'll ingest 220 calories or more if you go for the crackers or candy, but your "hunger" may be better satisfied for a longer period of time. On days when I indulge myself, I invariably eat much less the next day--not because I'm punishing myself, but because I've satisfied some physiological need for the junk food. Thus, if I splurge on 2200 calories one day, it balances out the next day when I may only eat 750.

A while back I had virtually no appetite for several days. It was hot and I was busy with projects, so I simply had no interest in eating more than 1,000 calories a day. At the end of the week, my husband and I took a six-mile day hike to a mountain lake. When we got back, I weighed myself to confirm my suspicions: I'd lost a lot of water weight and was the lowest I'd been since I was 14. That night, he and I went to a local eatery. I splurged my calories on a microbrew and a Mediterranean chicken wrap that came with a plate full of beer-battered french fries. After drinking half the beer, my willpower to resist the fries was gone. I ate them all with no regrets. It was all just splendid!

That night I suffered minor gas and indigestion from the greasy potatoes and flour tortilla wrap. But aside from a one-pound weight gain caused by water retention (the fries were salty), I was unscathed the next day and had surprisingly little appetite.   If I had been "good" and eaten only a bare salad for dinner, I'd probably have been obsessing the next day over the fries I could have had.   That, in turn, could lead me to a collapse of will over intellect, pushing me to binge just to "get even." So I was better off, in the long run, eating the fries.

Carrots, broccoli, spinach and kale are all good for me.   And I find them generally good-tasting. Yet, if my body doesn't crave them, I'm not going to substitute them for other foods just because they're healthy for me and will supposedly fill me up.   To do so would be to let my "intellect" (emotion) take over my eating decisions, and that's how I gained weight in the first place. Instead, I will listen to my body.   If the body needs it, the body will tell me.

BLWL Concept 9: "Keep it real"
Avoid "fake foods" because they appeal to the diet mentality.   Don't try to "fool" your body into thinking you've satisfied it with less than it really wants or needs.   Your body knows better!"

The most disgusting "food product" I've ever seen was a bag of so-called noodles that were supposedly made from some sort of plant fiber.   The company producing them claimed they had zero calories and zero nutrition, but they could be substituted for pasta in stroganoff and spaghetti.   The noodles resembled translucent tapeworms and had a foul smell when I opened the bag to heat them up.   A friend gave me the bag to try; she was thinking about becoming a distributor.   I told her what I thought of them and never heard any more about it. I'm assuming she changed her mind about investing in the company. I hope so.

She and many others had fallen prey to the idea that they could eat "fake foods" and feel satisfied. They could pretend they were eating old-fashioned egg noodles or creamy alfredo and "cheat" their minds into thinking it was the real thing. While you can cheat the mind for a short time, you can't cheat your body. It knows the difference between real food and fake.

Over the years I've tried to enjoy milkshakes made with powdered milk and ice. I've tried liquid meal replacements in cans, non-alcoholic beer, and "energy bars" made with stale grains, sugar and chemicals. With few exceptions, the "pretend" foods are void of taste and/or laden with so many chemical preservatives and artificial sweeteners that I wouldn't even feed them to a pet rat. Fake foods are an insult to your body and to your ability to lose or maintain weight. If an ingestible substance (I hate to call it "food") mimics a high calorie treat, you'll be tempted to eat way too much of it, and maybe even gorge on it, guilt-free. Eating with this mindset ("It's no calories, so I can gorge myself on it") is counter productive to the life-changing mindset necessary for sustained weight loss and maintenance. There is NO "real" food you can ever gorge on without paying consequences. To try to fool your body by eating these "fake foods" is just perpetuating a bad habit of eating without license. And it's an insult to the natural intelligence of your body.

If you want creamy fettuccine alfredo, eat a small amount of it. Eat as little of it as you can, enjoy it, and be satisfied with it. Honor your body and your true cravings with the real thing. Real food. Real nutrition. It will stick with you and satisfy you ten times better than anything that's fake.

BLWL Concept 10: "Lose the clock"
Don't eat a food, or eat at a certain time, just because others in your family are doing so. Your body is separate from theirs. So are your appetite and your metabolism. So is your life.

Our families and spouses expect us to sit down and enjoy meals with them, whether they cooked it, we cooked it, or we're eating out. It's a valuable ritual that fosters family togetherness and sharing. We should do everything possible to keep this ritual going, since it's so important to relationships.

But that doesn't mean we all have to eat the same thing. The ritual doesn't concern the type of food. It concerns the act of sitting down together to enjoy a meal or to share sustenance. That means you don't have to eat a portion of the eggs, bacon and hashbrowns if you don't want them. You can enjoy a piece of whole wheat bread, or a bowl of brown rice with almond milk and sweetener, or a hard-boiled egg without the bacon and hashbrowns. As long as you're sitting there, enjoying a meal, the ritual is being completed.

Be prepared for criticism and scrutiny from family members who scoff at your choices of breakfast foods while they gorge on the potatoes, bacon, and biscuits. Tune them out, shrug off their comments, smile and continue eating what you want. They will get used to seeing you eating brown rice, leftover salad, or even a couple pancakes while they wolf down the truly fattening stuff. Do not play into their hands by protesting about their comments. Learn to exercise nonchalance. Learn to ignore their comments or criticisms as if nothing meaningful was said (it wasn't), and take it with a grain of graceful composure. You are winning, and you will end up a role model for the rest of them!

BLWL Concept 11: "Water"
Drink as much water as you can stand. It is a wonder drug for weight loss and health.

There's something wrong with my mouth, I guess. I have a hard time gulping down liquids from a glass or mug. But stick a straw in it, and I'm ready to suck down gallons of liquid, be it a pitcher of margaritas, a cappuccino, or just plain water.

Just plain old water is the best of the three, of course, if you want to lose weight and feel healthy. The more the better. It is a magical elixir. You're not a heavy-duty water sot? Well, you might become one when you consider these benefits:

Water cleans out your mouth if you have a bad taste in it. In the past I tried to cover up bad tastes by eating something else. Now I know it's better to remove the taste with water than to cover it up with some other food. Heck, I even use it to get rid of really good tastes! My husband has a penchant for those peanut-butter-filled pretzels he gets in a big jug from Costco. If I occasionally stray too near the jug and snag one, I'll chase it down with about six ounces of water. If I leave the good taste lingering in my mouth, I'll be apt to dive into the jug for more of the same. I don't want to do that. Taste no evil, eat no evil.

Water fills you up. If you drink a couple glasses of water when you're hungry or craving, you literally don't have room in your stomach for much else. By the time you do, your craving may have passed.

Water will revive you better than any energy drink or power shot. It will wake you up and make you feel healthy instead of drugged. Try it some time when you're driving and you begin to feel drowsy. A few sips of cold water will do more for you than an Energy Shot, and it will be better for you than all those chemicals.

Water does wonders for the complexion. As you lose weight, you're going to have saggy skin. (Sorry about that, but believe me, it's worth it.) Keeping your skin well hydrated will minimize the sagginess and maintain elasticity. If you don't drink enough water while you're losing weight, you run the risk of looking like a meth addict. So pour that water into your system and plump up that radiant skin that's left behind after the fat departs for good.

Water is something you can drink any time, anywhere, and it's actually good for you. It's also cheap (or free if you don't require bottled water). If you need the snob appeal to really enjoy your drink, then go ahead and spring for a bottle of really expensive water from Switzerland or from ancient glaciers. Savor it like a fine wine. Brandish it in public. Enjoy the hell out of it. In reality, it's probably no better than your tap water at home, but if it makes you feel better drinking it, go for it! If, on the other hand, you want to go "on the cheap," most restaurants will give you a free glass of water with your meal. (They don't want you choking on the premises, after all). Some will even garnish with lemon if you request it. Do leave a commensurate tip if you get lemon.

Water doesn't stain your teeth like coffee or sugar-free cola. Our society is obsessed with the whiteness of our teeth. We spend millions a year on teeth-whitening toothpastes and treatments, to counteract what the coffee, tea, and colas to do our pearly-whites. Why not just forego the staining drinks and suck down the water instead? Ever tried hot water in a coffee mug or pretty teacup? I bet if you were sipping while you talked on the phone, you may not even notice that the liquid in your glass is clear and not brown. Remember that clear liquid equals whiter teeth.

Water keeps your breath fresh. As we age, our mouths often become dry. I notice a lot of my older friends chewing gum now. Gum is good, but water is better. Think of "dry mouth" as a signal that you need to drink more water. It will literally wash out your mouth and get rid of that horrid taste that gives us dragon-breath.

Water draws water out of your system. In other words, if you're retaining water, then drinking more water is the best thing you can do. Let's say you've been on a plateau; you haven't lost any weight for the past two weeks, despite your efforts to reduce caloric intake and to exercise more. Should you give up? **No! You should drink more water!** Your body is in a state of rebellion and is holding onto toxins that need to be flushed out. Who knows what sets it off! It could be the sodium in the rice pilaf mix you cooked up two nights ago. It could be hormones. It could be a change in weather, or seasonal allergies, or kidney malfunction, or a big reduction in your caloric intake. Obese people tend to retain more water than thin people. Your own water retention could be caused by a combination of these factors. Regardless, one thing is true: the water has to come out eventually. Drinking water, even when you're retaining it, is like priming the pump. It gets things moving. And no matter how uncomfortable you may feel drinking water when you're already "waterlogged," just remember there are NO calories in it!

Water rinses a lot of junk out of your body. It detoxifies your cells; it literally flushes out the bad stuff that causes you to retain weight. The research is out there, and it's sobering. If you drink two or less glasses of water a day, you have a 55% greater chance of developing colon cancer than people who drink more water. You also have a 79% greater chance of developing breast cancer if you limit your intake to two glasses of water a day.

Here's the bottom line: if you want to lose weight, stay healthy, and look good while you're doing it, you have to drink a lot of water. If you are otherwise reducing your caloric intake and increasing your caloric burn, and you're not losing weight, it's probably because you're not drinking enough water. Suck down a gallon of water over the next 24 hours and you'll see a chunk of weight fall off in the next couple days. Yes, it will be water. But it will be water laden with toxins and fat that have been clinging desperately to your organs for far too long.

How to get into the water habit:
Have a glass next to every sink in the house. Each time you pass the sink, drink at least half a glass.

Have water by your bedside. When you awaken with a dry mouth, have a sip of water.

Experiment with water temperature. You want water you can guzzle easily, without getting muscle contractions from the cold. Even if you've always chosen cold water, run the tap to about 80 degrees and try sucking down at least half a glassful. You just might find it more soothing and easier going down than the cold stuff.

Use straws. Most of us used straws when we were kids, and we tend to associate straws with kid drinks like Kool-Aid and soda fountain treats. Take that pleasant childhood association and stick it into a glass of water. Better yet, go to WalMart and buy a hot pink or lime green plastic insulated glass that has a straw built into the lid. Or take a cocktail glass, fill it with water, and stick a sipstick into it so you can pretend it's a fancy adult beverage. Straws offer a tidy way to mainline a beverage straight down your throat. They also give your mouth something to play with, and they're much lower in calories than pencils or peanuts.

Find a water bottle you absolutely love...one that fits your style and fits your purse or backpack...and carry it with you everywhere. Make a statement with it. I searched internet sites like Cafepress.com and Zazzle.com until I found the style and design that suited me. I figured if I found the perfect water bottle for me, I'd use it more. Mine had to have just the right kind of lid (leakproof in case I tipped it over), the right kind of spout (I like the little pull-up-to-open kind), the right size to fit in my car's beverage holder, and the right design so I could make a statement. Hey, it's an accessory, after all! My final choice: a cheap white plastic bottle that says in red letters, "I Kiss Pit Bulls!" I'm seldom seen without it these days.

When I'm served a glass of water in a restaurant, I ask them to "hold the ice" because my teeth are sensitive to the cold. You can certainly request your water any way you like it. Ask for water in a form that will be easy and pleasant for you to drink...and then drink it all before your meal arrives.

Keep a water bottle or sippy cup on your desk. When you have the urge to reach for a soda, reach for the water instead. You'll find it's an easy, pleasant, and very satisfying substitution. Often it's not *what* we're putting in our mouths, but the fact that we're just putting *something* in there.

Think of water as your friend....a friend you can't get enough of!

The biggest drawback to drinking lots of water is finding bathrooms. Yes, it takes some planning. But you'll also find your body adjusting so you won't have to pee quite so often as when you first start the increase in water consumption. Don't worry if you have to get up to pee once or twice in the night when you first start increasing your intake. It's your signal that you're drinking enough water. If you are healthy, your urine should be quite pale and almost odorless. If your urine is very yellow, and if it has a strong smell, you have a problem that needs to be addressed. You're probably dehydrated. Drink more water! Even though you don't feel thirsty, your body is crying out for liquids to flush itself. While concentrated urine can also be a sign of infection or uncontrolled diabetes, the most common reason is simply a lack of sufficient water.

Fill up your glass next time you pass the sink, and make a toast to the most miraculous liquid in the world. It's clean, refreshing, free, has no calories, no fat, no sodium, and no artificial coloring or flavor enhancers. It keeps your teeth white, your breath fresh, your stomach full, your skin from wrinkling, your joints from stiffening, and it gives you a longer, more enjoyable life. Cheers!

Chapter 10

• • • • • •

Q & A

1. My granddaughter is 16 and she wants to follow your program too. Is this okay for kids?

This book is intended for readers who are 40 and older. Kids shouldn't even be thinking about "bucket lists." Their bodies are still growing; they may not have even developed any food sensitivities yet. (I was 22 when I discovered I could no longer eat split pea soup without developing killer gas!) While some of my points are valid for anyone trying to maintain good health (like drinking lots of water and avoiding "fake foods"), I don't think young people should be going to bed hungry, weighing every day, or keeping close track of calories. It's up to us adults to set good examples for them by exercising and maintaining a healthful lifestyle.

2. I don't have any food sensitivity issues that I know of. I just like to eat!! What can I do about that?

First, ask yourself how you really feel. Are you sluggish? Moody? Easily fatigued? Stressed? Do your joints ache? Do you get headaches? Intestinal gas? Are your elimination habits irregular? Do you get cravings for certain foods? Are you sleepy at work? Do you have trouble sleeping at night? Do you have trouble getting out of bed in the morning? Do you think there may be a connection between these symptoms and your eating habits? I certainly do!

Sadly, many people don't even know what "feeling good" feels like. Their "normal" usually includes at least some of the above symptoms. Imagine for a moment...you're pain-free, calm, contented yet energized. Your gut is quiet--not full or bloated. It's easy to breathe. Stretching feels good. It doesn't hurt to stand up. You bounce up a flight of stairs like you're eight years old. You sleep soundly at night and wake up ready to jump out of bed and start the day. Your mind is clear. You're self-assured, confident and capable. You're physically as strong as you need to be. Your joints move freely. Your mind feels at total peace residing within your body.

Contrast that picture to this one: you crawl out of bed needing a cup of coffee to get going. The coffee leaves you with a trace of heartburn, so you chase it down with a bagel. At mid-morning you're still thinking about that bagel, and your stomach is grumbling, so you grab a donut. At lunch you realize you really should eat something "healthful," so you have a banana. By mid-afternoon you're feeling sleepy and just a tad gassy. You need something to wake you up and give you a lift, so you eat a small bag of Skittles. That helps for about an hour, and then you begin to crash again. Now you're starting to feel cranky, and that brings an onset of hip and knee discomfort. There must be something you can eat to make yourself feel better! Maybe a couple pieces of cheddar cheese and a cocktail before dinner. The cocktail makes you feel much better, of course! For dinner you're serving steak, fried potatoes and salad to your spouse. Normally you wouldn't eat potatoes, but the one little piece you tried was so good that you have a few more, and end up eating all the leftovers.

If this sounds even vaguely familiar, you probably have food sensitivities you should heed. It may have started with the bagel; its carbohydrates triggered a sensation of extreme hunger. The donut was available, so you grabbed that and perpetuated the gluten/carbohydrate/hunger cycle. The banana was probably a good choice, although it may have worked in consort with the gluten to produce mild gassiness. The Skittles, made from high fructose corn syrup, sugar and food dye, gave you a fast charge followed by a crash that felt like a mild hangover. Because you feel crappy now, you're cranky. Everything seems worse, including the inflammation throughout your body. The cheese was good, until you ate the second piece which landed in your gut like lead. The cocktail removed all your inhibitions, making it okay for you to eat the potatoes, which you know darn well do not agree with you. Needless to say, you went to bed feeling somewhat "heavy" and suffering a mild headache. You wake up and start the whole cycle all over again.

Moral of the story: You do have food sensitivities. Once you start paying closer attention to how certain food interactions affect you, you're on your way to feeling truly good, perhaps for the first time in your life.

3. I hate drinking water.

Tough. Get used to it. Water keeps you alive. Drinking water is probably the single most respectful thing you can do to honor your body. Besides that, it has absolutely no drawbacks. So grab your water bottle and start sucking. Rather than go through the regimentation of measuring how much you drink each day, just get the habit of drinking water at every opportunity. Every. Opportunity.

4. The charts say I should weigh 150. I think that's too much.

If you're not comfortable with your body at 150, go lower. Between charts, internet advice, doctors, family and friends, you'll find a lot of varying opinions. The bottom line is how you feel, physically and emotionally. You'll know when you get there. My Wii Fit program tells me that 148.6 is the ideal weight for someone my height and age, because it's the weight at which I'm most able to fend off illness. It wasn't satisfactory to me, so I've chosen to hover around 140. I keep wondering if I couldn't lose another couple pounds, but then I see pictures of myself, slip into my Size 6 jeans with ease, and realize that I really am where I want to be. *When you no longer feel one bit self conscious about your size, you have reached your goal.*

5. The charts say I should weigh 150. I think that's too low.

I used to think the same thing. "I'll look emaciated, like a cancer victim, at that weight," I told myself. But when the weight started to steadily come off as a result of my *BLWL* lifestyle changes, I realized I had much more to lose than I'd ever imagined. Can you feel your hipbones? If not, you have more weight on you than you need. Reprogram yourself to be truly thin. Provided you're staying healthy, lose as much weight as you can. Don't stop at your usual stopping place of a 15-pound weight loss. Keep going. It's not a 10K road race, it's a 26-mile marathon! Push yourself into that unknown territory of lightness and thinness you may not have experienced since you were a teenager. You can absolutely get there! And by the time you're there, you'll stay there because you're not dieting; you've simply changed the way you do things. Forever.

6. Where do I get a Wii Fit, and how much does it cost?

You need the basic Nintendo Wii console first. Check the big-box stores and electronics centers, plus eBay, Craig's List, and other online stores. Prices will vary from around $60 to $200, depending on what extras are included. I got mine off eBay for about $70. The Wii Fit package (balance board and software) came from a second-hand store: $50. If you buy the Wii Fit (now called Wii Fit Plus) new, it may run around $140. Wherever you buy a Wii console, you should also be able to find the Wii Fit Plus package. Often the package will include extra software with more Wii sports games. Shop around.

7. What about that extra skin?

I do have a lot of baggy skin. It shocks me sometimes, but it doesn't really bother me. I am, after all, no longer a spring chicken. I spent way too much time in the sun when I was younger. And I've lost nearly 25 percent of my body mass. That all adds up to a lot of sagginess on my otherwise well-muscled arms and around my tummy. But clothing hides it! Not that I'm ashamed of it. To me, it's an indication of success at something I've wanted all my life to achieve. Feeling 30 years younger than my age and wearing a Size 6 are well worth a bit of baggy skin.

8. What are the best, most inspirational diet books you've read?

The Story of Weight Watchers (A Signet Book), by Jean Nidetch, 1979.

Diets Don't Work, by Bob Schwartz, 2002.

9. I don't have any self discipline like you do. I can't do this.

BLWL isn't about self discipline! It's about choosing to make changes that make you feel better. When you know you have a life-threatening reaction to shell fish, it's an easy choice to not eat them. When you know that red wine gives you a headache, it's easy to choose white instead. When you know that eating certain foods will cause a negative reaction in your body later, it's easy to avoid them. It's a matter of slowing down and thinking before we put something in our mouths. The old adage, "A moment on the lips, forever on the hips" comes to mind, even when we're thinking about indigestion, aches and pains. We only enjoy food for that fleeting moment we're eating it. We pay the price for hours or days. The short pleasure we get from eating certain foods isn't worth the long-lasting discomfort we feel later.

You can do this, just as I have. As soon as you start feeling truly good, you will have seen the light. Simply follow it.

10. I'm so confused. There are so many diets, and all my friends have their own strong opinions about what works and what doesn't.

Diets don't work because they are designed to be temporary. Pay no attention to your friends when they're raving about the newest diet fad. You are as much, or more of, an expert on this subject than any of them. Look at any of your friends or acquaintances who have lost significant amounts of weight and kept it off for many years. They made lifestyle changes. They didn't finally lose the weight for good by taking injections, fasting, or eating pre-packaged meals. They took steps they were willing to incorporate into their everyday lives, for the rest of their lives. They did it to feel better overall, not to be able to squeeze into a smaller size for the upcoming class reunion.

11. I'm afraid to lose the weight because I'm afraid I'll gain it back. This is the great thing about *Bucket List Weight Loss*. As the name implies, this is the last time you'll ever have to worry about losing weight. You accomplish your goal, and you stay there, because your eating and exercise habits are permanently changed. For decades I lived with the same fear of gaining back weight once I'd lost 15 or 20 pounds on a crash diet. Generally, when people start diets, it's with a short-term goal in mind. Long-term, permanent changes are not addressed. Of course, the assumption is always, "If I start to gain it back, I'll just fall back on the crash diet program for a few days again." But that's the yo-yo in motion, and your body learns to resist those big boomerangs while it gradually increases to ever-greater proportions. However, with *Bucket List Weight Loss*, you're not dieting; you are, instead, making changes that you will want to live with for the rest of your life. The weight won't come back.

12. Should I be professionally tested for food sensitivities?

If you can afford it, the results may prove enlightening. However, listening to your body's reactions to certain problematic foods will give you a pretty darn good feel for what you should and shouldn't be including in your diet. I have no idea whether or not I have full-blown Celiac Disease. I doubt I do, since I occasionally fall off the wagon and eat some gluten, and the results are uncomfortable but not severe. I just know I feel better when I avoid gluten, and I don't need a professional test to prove it.

13. My best friend says I shouldn't lose any more weight, but I think I still need to lose 10 more pounds.
Beware the friend who may have 10 pounds (or more) to lose and tells you that you've lost "enough." You're the only person who knows where you're comfortable. Don't let other people sabotage your intentions with their placations of "Oh, be careful not to lose too much!" It's considered, in many circles, the "thing to say." It implies that they never thought you were very overweight to begin with, or that they don't think you can lose it anyway.

14. What about anorexia? Am I at risk of becoming anorexic on this plan?

While it is a disturbing fact that anorexia has, in recent years, become an issue with older adults and not just teenage girls, the chances of you developing anorexia are slim if you keep in mind your *Bucket List Weight Loss* is meant to improve your overall health, not diminish it. Your health, and how you feel, are your yardsticks here for measuring how thin you should become.

15. What's your own biggest stumbling block?

Alcohol. I love my adult beverage in the evening. Since I'm unwilling to give up alcohol, that means I have to budget about 250 calories each day just for that. The hidden danger with alcohol, for me, is the way it melts my resistance and clouds my judgment when it comes to eating later on. With disgusting nonchalance, I can turn that 250-calorie liquid treat into 900 calories or more, just because I end up eating more of the wrong things when I'm drinking.

16. Is life really perfect when you're as skinny as you want to be? Life improves dramatically when you're thin and healthy, but it's still just life. You'll have days of depression and frustration, and you'll be tempted to eat irresponsibly to make it better. But remember, that kind of eating will just compound your misery and spiral you right into a pit. Accept the fact that some days you're just going to be miserable, and food used like a drug will only make it worse.

17. How do I eat out and still keep with the program?
If you're talking about once a day, change your habits and start carrying your own food with you for lunch. If you're talking about once a week, don't worry about it. Eat what you want, as long as you ask your body for permission and remember the effects you will

feel four hours later. You will automatically begin to balance out your days between feasts and famines, so to speak. If you eat too much at the restaurant, you will probably eat substantially less the next day because you will still be satisfied from last night's meal. Of course, you might find yourself leaning more toward salads the next time you eat out, and you'll probably opt out on the breadsticks and maybe even the salad dressing. I seldom use dressing on my salads anymore because I've come to enjoy the taste of the actual vegetables instead of covering them up with a bunch of processed white goo. This was a natural evolution for me. One day I just realized I liked my salads better with just a little salt and pepper. Don't be surprised if your tastes evolve the same way.

18. Should I check with my doctor before starting this program?

If you have pre-existing medical issues, or if you think you might, then you'd better check with your doctor first. I'm supposed to tell you that anyway, so consider it done.

19. You say I should listen to my gut. My gut wants donuts at 11 a.m., Taco Bell for lunch, a bag of chips and a soda for dinner, followed by half a package of cookies before bed and a couple more when I get up at 2:30 a.m.

You can't know what your gut is asking for until the given time, so don't predict what it will want later in the day. And listen more closely. Is it your gut asking for donuts, or is it your mind? Your gut is a finely designed machine. It probably wants something but it's not really asking for a greasy, sticky wad of dough made with bleached white flour and void of nutrients. If it's growly, it could probably stand a couple swigs of water. If it feels unsettled, maybe some yogurt will help. It's the mind that's pushing the donuts, just like a street corner thug pushing drugs. Remember what drugs do. Remember what donuts do. You'll crash and feel horrible after either one.

Make yourself a list of healthful, reasonably low-fat foods that you enjoy so much they're like treats to you. Eliminate the ones that are overprocessed and laden with sodium. Eliminate the ones you suspect may trigger cravings for other things. Now stock up on those foods. When you feel the need to eat, grab one of them. I'm not talking celery sticks and carrots. I'm talking rice crackers, hommus, Greek yogurt, grapes, brown rice, cooked chicken breasts, lean burgers, berries, artichokes, sunflower nuts, olives, almonds, eggs, edamame. Whole foods that have their individual tastes and textures. Season them if you want; dress them up with bacon bits, parmesan cheese, olive oil, salt and pepper, dried cranberries and dried blueberries (or fresh if you can get them!) You'll be shocked at how wonderful these individual foods start to taste, and how satisfying they are, once your body has weaned itself off chemicals, preservatives and sodium. They will be your go-to foods when your stomach says, "Feed me!"

20. I'm too damn tired to exercise after a busy day. All I want to do is stop at Burger King and get something to bring home.

Stop at Burger King and get a large diet soda at the drive-up window. Then drive home, think about the food you can snag as soon as you get there (see the above suggestions). Drink a large glass of water when you get home, and then turn on the TV while you grab a container of Greek yogurt, rip the lid off it, squirt in some agave nectar, give it a stir, and dive into it with a big spoon while you settle in to watch TV. Eat as much of it as you like. The whole giant container only has 560 calories (plain, fat-free). Oh yes…add about 50 calories for the agave nectar. Polish off your diet soda, if you haven't already. Burp. Think about whether or not your stomach is hungry anymore. Believe me, it isn't. If you feel tempted to go back to

Burger King at 10:00, go to bed instead. It's dangerous out there, and people will think you're really weird if they see you ordering a big meal at the drive-thru, by yourself, that late at night.

21. What about eating low-cal, low-fat foods? Shouldn't I always be looking for those? Eat them only if you truly enjoy them, but don't try to substitute something tasteless (like low-fat cheese) when your digestive system is telling you it actually desires the fat found in cheddar. If you're trying to decide between snacking on a Golden Delicious apple or a green pepper, don't choose the green pepper just because it's lower in calories. Eat what will satisfy you and what tastes good. If you want to make popcorn, look at the calorie difference between the "lite" and the "real butter." Chances are you'll choose the "lite." But if you must have butter, go ahead. Just budget it into your daily calories. Sugar-free Jello is fine if you really want dessert, but you're better off learning to just stop eating before it's time for dessert. Remember that you no longer have to eat anything at a certain time, just because you've always done it that way.

22. My doctor told me several small meals a day is better than one or two big ones, but you're saying it's okay to go all day without eating if I'm not hungry.

There's a difference between conscious "fasting" and simply not eating because you're neither hungry nor interested in food. Your doctor is right in saying your body runs most efficiently if it always has a small amount of food in the stomach. Your blood sugar remains even that way, and your organs are less stressed. But if your hunger level is only around 4 on a scale of 1 to 10, don't eat unless you think you won't get the opportunity later on when you'll need the fuel. For example, if it's 6:00 in the evening and I haven't eaten anything since 4:00, and I'm not hungry, I may not eat anything more before I go to bed. I won't need any extra energy to help me make it through a night of sleep. But if my stomach has been empty since I woke up, and I'm planning a strenuous afternoon of dog training or yard work, I'm going to eat something to prevent myself from crashing in the middle of my activities. Rather than eat a big, greasy breakfast or a heavy lunch, I'll grab a hard-boiled egg, some Greek yogurt, or some seedless red grapes. That, combined with plenty of water for sipping, will be more than enough to get me through the afternoon without light-headedness. In the evening, I may have a piece of chicken at 5:00, a killer spinach salad at 6:30, and a cup of yogurt an hour later. That's three to five small meals. That should keep your doctor happy and your body even happier.

23. My coworkers are constantly sabotaging me by bringing goodies to work...or wanting to have lunch "out" all the time. How do I deal with this?

You're programmed to accept their goodies, to eat food when it's in sight, and to join in the camaraderie of lunch "out." You think it would be rude to decline their offers and to pass on their brownies and cookies. There's joy in sharing good food and there's company in the misery you all feel after you eat too much of a good thing.

Just because everyone else is parachuting out of a perfectly good airplane doesn't mean you have to do the same. Here are some ways you can handle situations like this in the future:

1. Tell them you have diarrhea. They won't want you anywhere near their food.

2. Thank them graciously and accept the box of cupcakes your client brought you. Then take them to the break room and leave them there for coworkers. They'll disappear.

3. Thank them graciously but explain that you're being allergy tested for gluten, sugar, chocolate, dairy, or whatever else they're offering you, so you have to decline the goodies.

4. If someone wants to take you to a fast-food lunch place, tell them you brought your own. (Besides, do you have any idea what you SMELL like when you come back from lunch at a place like that? Ugh!)

5. If someone wants to take you to a nice place for lunch, order a big salad and enjoy it--without dressing! (Yes, that really is possible!)

There's a lot to be said for keeping temptation out of your path, especially when you're first starting to learn new eating habits. See no goodies, eat no goodies. Get them away from your line of sight. Don't go to restaurants where smells and sights will tempt you and cause you to feel so sorry for yourself that you cave in and over-eat. As your body adjusts and starts communicating more forcefully with your mind, those temptations will cease to exist. You won't even want one of those brownies. Ice cream won't interest you. The mere thought of french fries will give you cramps. Until then, isolate yourself from them.

24. I LOVE diet pop. How long does it take to feel better when you QUIT drinking diet pop? I get headaches and feel horrible....like coming off a drug.

You don't have to quit drinking diet sodas! But if you're drinking more than two a day, you might want to cut down when you learn that:

- The phosphates in them are bad for your bones.

- The sodium will cause serious water (weight) retention.

- The combination of sodium and caffeine can be dehydrating, which means you'll want to drink more (like drinking seawater because the seawater you just drank made you thirstier).

- *You are 57% more likely to gain weight if you drink a lot of diet soda.* I know, it doesn't seem to make sense on the surface. But many years of repeated studies have proven a correlation between drinking diet sodas and gaining weight. The sodas themselves don't make you obese, but they trigger something internally that tells us we must eat more. The body has a way of knowing when you're fooling it. If you fill it with artificially sweetened crap of zero nutritional value, your body will go on alert searching for the real thing. That equates to cravings, which usually leads to overeating. So you actually end up consuming many more calories at the end of the day than you would have if you'd just stuck to water, tea, or something without artificial sweeteners.

I don't have anything against artificial sweeteners when used in moderation to rev up something bland like plain yogurt. My biggest problem with diet drinks--or anything processed, for that matter--is the sodium. It will cause water retention, which slows your weight loss--which is depressing and discouraging--which can lead to giving up--which can lead to overeating--which can lead to weight gain, not loss. So if you give sodium a free rein, whether it's in your diet soda or your Rice-A-Roni, it can end up making you fatter.

Try substituting healthier drinks and backing off the diet soda. Get flavored iced teas, or add a drink powder like Crystal Lite to a bottle of water. Do check the sodium levels on the labels, as they will vary. Walmart makes a good powdered drink mix that's practically sodium free. Always opt for low-sodium or sodium-free if you can.

If you enjoy the carbonation of diet sodas, get your bubblies from seltzer water or club soda. (Note: seltzer is just carbonated water, whereas club soda contains sodium.) You can also buy a countertop soda/sparkling water machine and add your own flavorings. Even if your homemade concoctions contain a little sugar, you can still cut out the high fructose corn syrup, sodium benzoate, and artificial food colorings that come in store-bought sodas. Doesn't that just sound better?

The headaches come from your physical dependence on the sodium and caffeine in the drinks. If you stopped your "coke habit" cold turkey, you might have about three days of flu-like withdrawal symptoms: headache, nausea, shakes, muscle and joint discomfort, and definitely crankiness. None are life-threatening. The more water you drink, and the busier you stay during this time, the faster you'll recover. It's like being "functionally hung over," at worst. It will pass.

25. They say that exercise will give you "energy." It does NOT do that for me. How long do you have to exercise religiously before you will start to notice a change...and actually feel energized from it?

If you're more than 50 pounds overweight, movement isn't much fun at first. You're fighting your bodyweight with every step you take and every move you make. That fight can leave you exhausted before you've accomplished much. So start slowly, maybe with a walk around the block, or a half-hour Leslie Sansone "Walk Away the Pounds" video workout. Do it twice a day and your mind will start looking forward to it *on the third day.* By the fourth day, your body will be asking you for it. Then it's just a matter of keeping your momentum going, and maybe lengthening or varying your workout. Never work to the point of exhaustion. Always end your workout before your body starts screaming obscenities at you. The exercise should be a treat to your body, not a punishment.

The "energy" you feel from movement is caused by increased and improved blood flow and circulation. In fact, all your internal organs work better (and feel better) because they're getting more blood and more oxygen. That alone will give you energy. Exercise also releases endorphins (natural feel-good drugs) from your brain. Endorphins stimulate your metabolism and help your muscles grow, all of which makes you feel younger and healthier.

If you're not feeling an energy boost from moving your body, you're not doing the right kind of exercise. Remember it's not punishment; it should be enjoyable. How can a person not enjoy walking through a beautiful park on a warm summer evening or a crisp fall afternoon? Get your mind involved; smell autumn leaves, catch a snowflake on your tongue, count the daffodils coming up in the spring, and just think about how good it is to be alive and able to move. Listen to music or an audio book, or mentally plan your next vacation. Exercise is as much for the mind as it is for the body. Feel like a kid again…or just act like one. Whether you're walking, dancing, riding a bike or rowing a boat, think of your exercise as "play."

If you have a substantial layer of fat over your muscles, don't expect to *see* any popeye bulges until you lose the fat. That doesn't mean the muscles aren't firming up and working for you. As your muscles become more stretched and toned through *movement* (aka exercise), your joints will feel better because muscles are now supporting them. They're hugging your joints and protecting them. How can any of that not make you feel more energized?

26. I buy boxes of 100-calorie snacks so I can have something small as a treat. The problem is, I can't stop at just one package.....I can eat the whole box of treats because I know they're there.

First, let's look at what's typically in those 100-calorie snack packs: processed flour, refined sugar, salt, hydrogenated fat, and chemicals to color and preserve those fine ingredients. Whether you're eating 100 calories of cookies, 100 calories of cheese crackers, or 100 calories of chex mix, you're eating garbage that will probably trigger cravings a few minutes later, start a low-grade inflammation throughout your body, and cause you to retain water. So that kind of junk is an insult to your body to begin with, and it initiates a chain reaction of other unpleasantries that wreck your weight-loss efforts.

Second, the 100-calorie idea works best for people who don't have access to the rest of the carton throughout the day. You take 100 calories in your lunchbox, or you take 100 calories in your backpack. In theory, if you're at work or school, you don't have access to more than you brought with you, so you learn to "make do" with the 100-calorie pack. But once again, the real problem is the lack of nutritional value in these snacks. They'll hit the bottom of your stomach, and ten minutes later you won't even know they're in there. You won't feel satisfied. You'll only want more.

The 100-calorie packs are a clever marketing ploy for unsuspecting and well-intentioned dieters and snackers. Every time I see someone put a box of those in their Costco shopping cart, I think, "What a sucker."

Give away the ones you have left, and don't buy any more!

27. I can't do this.

That's just plain silly. I am not special. Neither are you. I did it.
I am you. Now you do it.

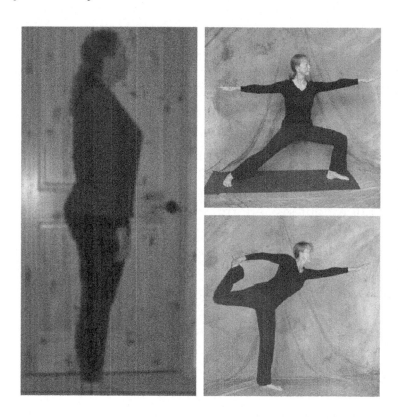

An afterthought...
for men only

Guys, let me tell you the cold, hard facts. There is nothing sexy or physically appealing about a fat gut that hangs over a belt. Is that blunt enough?

Call me a bitch, but I'm telling you the truth. You form your instant opinions about us women based on our boob and butt sizes. You talk about us, you look, you point, you chuckle. That's natural and we understand that. Which is part of the reason we're so hell-fired determined to make ourselves look good. If we're going to be talked about, we want it to be complimentary, even if it's crude.

It may be a surprise to you, but the ball bounces in both directions. Women tend to be a bit more reserved about such things--especially women in the 50-and-over category. But we notice. We fantasize. We lust, just like you. And we definitely do not lust over the thought of being crushed beneath a huge mass of naked, jiggling bellyfat while you pant and wheeze. Yes, we really do wonder what would happen if our big, fat men died of a heart attack, in bed, on top of us. That is not a sexy thought. In fact, it's a bigtime turn-off.

I remember, with a shudder, the first time I ever saw a man with "Dunlaps Disease" (where the stomach "done laps over" the belt) take his clothes off. I was aghast to see the stomach that had been "up there" fall to "down there." Somehow I thought the man would have the same basic shape when he removed his belt, but of course he didn't. The 30-year-old man aged about 30 more years right before my eyes. He had the physique of Elmer Fudd, whom I don't think is sexually attractive.

The real reason we don't like our own men fat: we don't want you to die! We love you, and we know that statistically we'll probably outlive you. You're likely to die of heart disease and related conditions that can be directly connected to obesity. We don't like that. We know it doesn't need to be that way, and we don't understand why living longer, healthier and sexier isn't important enough to you to make the necessary changes. We're retired or at least heading rapidly in that direction, and we want to enjoy those golden years with you guys, not with a bunch of golden girls in a Florida condo.

Please, please do this for us! Lose the extra 50 pounds you're carrying around your midsection. Quit trying to fool yourself (or us) into thinking it's muscle. We know better. Give us the gift of a few more years with you. Make your bodies physically attractive to us again, or at least make an effort for us. Heck, do it for yourself. You have nothing to gain but more years, more youthfulness, more physical ability to enjoy your favorite sports, and more sex.

Good physiques turn us on. Big bellies turn us off. Don't force us to keep faking it!

###

Bucket List Weight Loss Recap

1. Think four hours ahead. How will your gut feel? How will your mind and joints feel? Will you be gassy? Remember the "hangover principle." If you don't want to feel the bad effects later, avoid the food now.

2. If you're depressed and feeling miserable or angry, you'll be even worse off if you eat because of it. If you do NOT eat, you may still be depressed and angry...but you will also be THINNER...and thus, you'll feel much better.

3. Go to bed hungry. You will fall asleep and wake up not hungry and THINNER. The growlier your stomach is at bedtime, the better you will feel in the morning.

4. Keep a running tally of your calories. You'll find no need to "throw in the towel" for the day just because you fell off the wagon and ate three cookies. You may still be well within your range of 1000-1200 calories a day.

5. Move! Keep your body in the perpetual motion it seeks.

6. Weigh EVERY day to keep yourself on track and to learn about (and to accept) your body's natural fluctuations.

7. Converse with and listen to your body, not your mind. Does your body tell you it really wants and/or needs to eat right now? If not, don't eat. Tell the mind to shut up.

8. Don't eat something just because it's good for you. If your body doesn't want it at the moment, don't eat it. Either eat NOTHING, or eat what your body really tells you it wants/ needs.

9. Avoid "fake foods." Don't try to "fool" your body into thinking you've satisfied it with less than it really wants or needs. Your body knows better!

10. Don't eat a food, or eat at a certain time, just because others in your family are doing so. Your body is independent of theirs.

11. Drink as much water as you can stand. It is a wonder drug for weight loss and health.

About the author

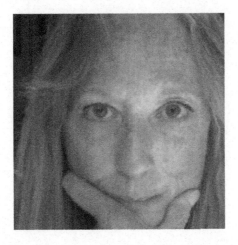

Jan Manning's articles have been published in more than 200 periodicals, ranging from *Christian Single* to *Cosmopolitan* to *Soldier of Fortune*. <u>*Bucket List Weight Loss*</u> is her first published full-length work.

Since retiring to her dream home in Montana, she's tried to make time for the activities she loves most: cross-country skiing, horse-back riding, and lake kayaking. But ideas for new writing projects keep interfering.

Connect with Jan Manning on-line:

https://www.facebook.com/jan.o.manning

http://www.bucketlistweightloss.com

Made in the USA
Monee, IL
27 April 2022

95536915R00085